The Ultimate Guide To DIY Homemade Medical Face Mask:

(Both Making Reusable Face Mask With Ear Savers, Filter Pockets, Without Elastic Band And No Sewing Method And How To Clean + Reuse Your Face Mask)

Table of Content

Introduction

In the period of disease epidemic, wearing of Face mask has become a social responsibility and as a means to curb the spread of disease especially respiratory syncytial virus. There are other preventive measures to take such as frequent washing of hands, avoid touching your face, mouth and eyes, spraying disinfectant around your environment, using hand sanitizer with at least 60% alcohol when washing of hand is not available, maintaining social distancing at least six feet away especially from a sick person, avoiding crowded environment.

What exactly is Face Mask?

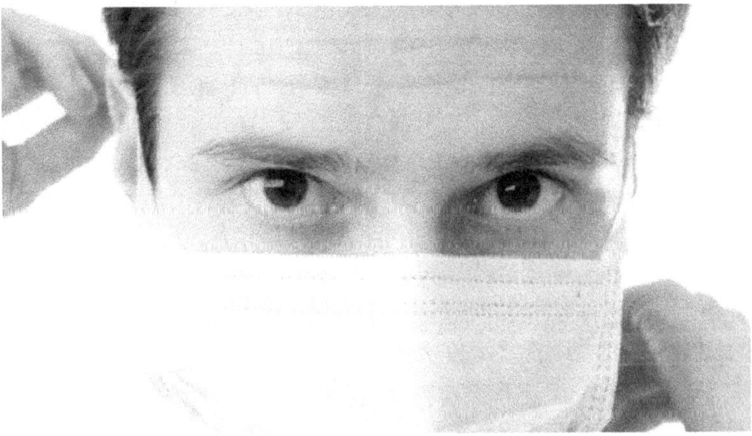

Face masks are snug fitting masks that cover the

nose and mouth area of your face and may have either ear loops or string ties or elastic bands to hold firm at the back of the head. Facemasks aid to reduce the spread of germs. If a person talks, coughs, or sneezes they release tiny liquid droplet into the atmosphere around them that can infect others. If a sick person wears a facemask, it helps to reduce the quantity of bacteria or virus droplets the person releases and can protect other people from becoming sick. A face mask also protects the person who wears it from being contaminated by nose and mouth splashes or sprays of body fluids.

There are varieties of facemask based on their quality, materials and sealed nature and they come in different colors. It is important to use a face mask approved by the CDC, WHO and FDA. we have the respirators face mask such as N95, FFP mask which are designed to protect more effectively against the air borne diseases due to the nature of their material, shape and tight seal. We also have a pre cast form fitting type of facemask, this is customized to fit the client face. They are made from thin fiber and can filter out tiny particle when wearing them. They are very expensive. We have the medical or surgical face mask which are mostly worn by medical professional during surgery or nursing. And meant to reduce the chance spreading airborne disease and other communicable diseases to others and prevent the breathing in of airborne dust particles, virus and bacteria. though they are less effective compared to respirators, but they can filter up to 90% of these tiny particles if made with good quality filters

In early sixties, the medical facemask were made from non-woven fabrics that are created through a melting blown process.it is usually a three ply material with the melt blown polymer usually polypropylene acting as the filter place between the non-woven fabric to prevent microbes from entering or leaving the mask .pleat are used to add elasticity to the mask such that the mask can expand to cover form the nose to the chin and then secured to the head with ear loops or elastic bands   but now the material is being replaced by cloth fabric as the N95 became scarce due to high demand and as the polymer material are in shortage . the CDC approved the use of cloth face coverings as mask or using cloth fabric to make medical face masks. Which can be washed and reuse.

Proper ways to put on and remove a face mask

Disposable face masks are meant to be used only in one cycle and then trashed. Except where getting another one is impossible then you may need to check out later in this book alternative ways of sterilizing and reusing your used mask because in times of epidemic having a mask is better than nothing You are required also to remove and replace masks when they become moist.

How to put on a face mask

1.   first of all wash your hands with soap and water or hand sanitizer if water and soap are not available before touching the mask.

2.   inspect the mask to ensure that there are no tears or holes on any side of the mask.

3.   check to see which side of the mask the top is. The side of the mask that has a stiff bendable edge is the top and is meant to fit snugly on your nose.

4.   identify the side of the mask that should be the front. Usually it is colored and brighter than the other side of the mask. you must wear it facing away from you, while the other side which is usually soft touches your face.

5   If you are using a Face Mask with Ear loops: just place each of the loop around your ear.

        For Face Mask that are made with string Ties: lower the mask such that it is at your nose

level and tie the mask over the crown of your head
and knot it.

Face Mask made with elastic Bands: use your
fingertips to hold the top of the mask and let the e
headbands to hang freely below your hands
position the mask to be at the same level with
your nose and pull the top strap over your head so
that it rests over the crown of your head. Do the
same with the bottom strap such that it rests at
the nape of your neck.

6.   ensure that it snugly fit around the nose
area.

7.   If using a face mask with ties: Then take the
bottom ties, one in each hand, and make a knot to
secure it at the nape of your neck.

8.   let the bottom part of the mask cover your
mouth and chin.

Correct way to remove a face mask

1.   wash your hands with soap and water or
hand sanitizer where the former is not available
before removing the mask. Avoid making contact
with the front of the mask. It may be
contaminated. He safe place to touch should be the
ear loops/ties/band. Follow the Removal methods
below according to the type of mask you are using.

2.   Face Mask with Ear loops: Hold both ear
loops and gently lift and remove the mask.

3.   Face Mask with Ties: Untie the bottom knot
before untying the top knot, then you can now pull
the mask away from you to remove it.

4.   Face Mask with Bands: starting from the bottom strap pull it over your head then pull the top strap off.

5.   Throw the mask in the trash if it is a disposable one and quickly wash your hands with soap and water or sanitize your hand.

The Correct Way to Wear A Cloth Face Mask or Covering

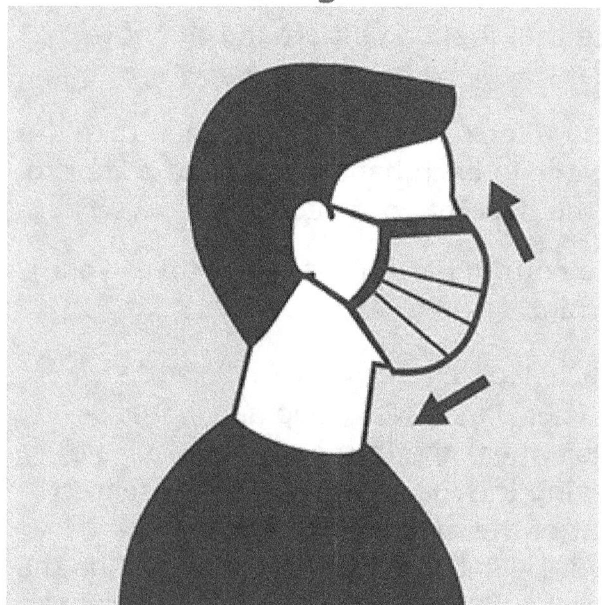

Cloth face mask or covering

- Should fit well especially around the nose area giving comfort around the side of the face
- it should be made secured with ties or ear loops
- it should include 2- 3 layers of fabric

- it must be made of breathable material which allows for breathing with no restriction
- it should be washable and easy to dry without damage or change to shape or material

☐

DIY Homemade Medical Face Mask

 In this book, we are going to be learning how to make effective medical face mask with ear savers, with or without elastic band , sewing methods , non-sewing methods , with make shift filters like heap vacuum bag   and also how to clean and re use them . so let dive in right away

Medical Face mask with HEPA Filter Vacuum Bag

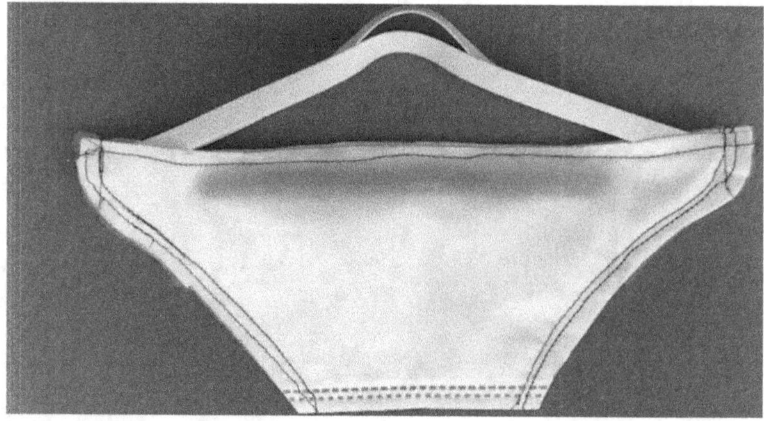

 This face mask is best used by health workers where there are shortage of   medical face mask and N95 respirators and it is the best home made face mask that is close to N95 face mask as they are more effective than the cloth fabric face mask that still allows virus to penetrate because   cotton which is the main material used on cloth covering face mask cannot prevent virus from penetrating the mask, it only allows you not to spread your own fluids or droplet to others But HEPA filter vacuum bag is an OSHA certified standard material that has the capacity to filters out 99.97% of airborne particulate matter according to the osha standards. It is also recommended by the CDC in their current publication to be considered as a home-made face mask material where there is no or shortage of N95 respirators especially when caring for a sick person with Covid -19, tuberculosis, measles and varicella

Precautions :

- Before making these masks ensure that you are not sick yourself so that you do not produce a contaminated face mask
- Ensure that you wash your hands with soap and water before you proceed.
- Store or distribute this mask in a clean and sanitized Ziplock bag to avoid contamination

Materials

- HEPA filter vacuum bag
- Glue gun with a glue stick
- Two pieces of elastic band 6 inches each (or rubber bands, string, cloth strips, or hair ties)
- Needle and thread (or bobby pin)
- Scissors
- Sewing machine
- Pencils and pipe cleaner

- A Template that you can download that shows a standard regular size face mask

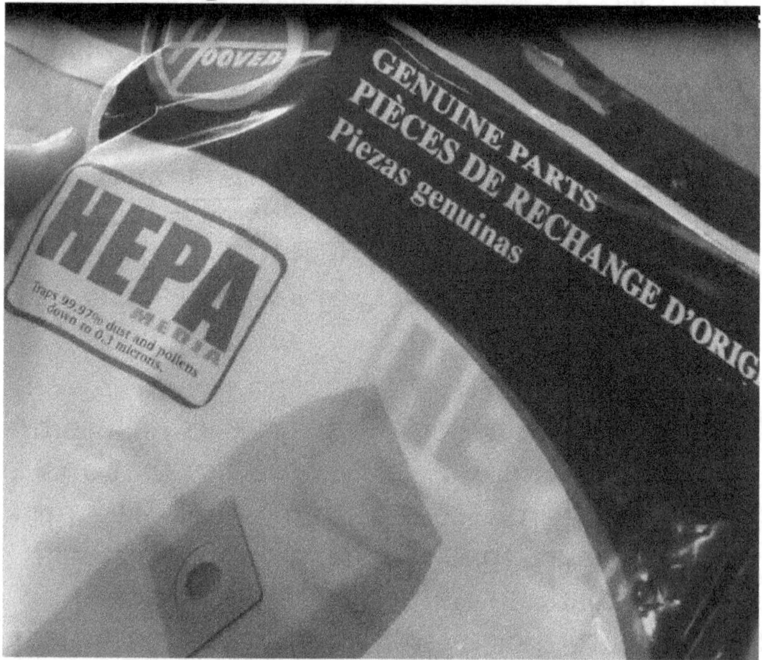

-
- Hepa vaccum bag

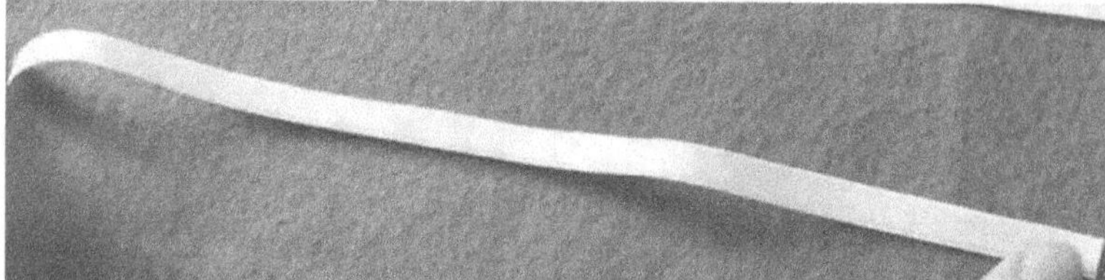

-
- Two of these elastic band

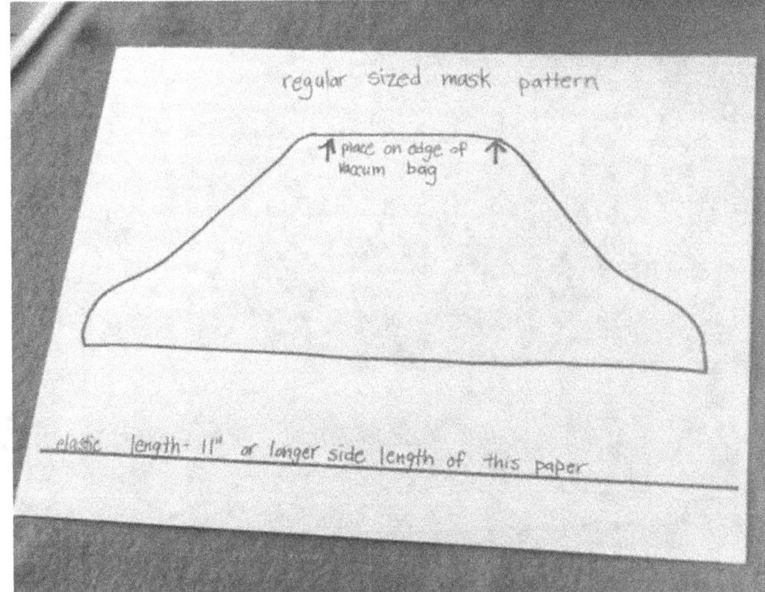

-
- Regular size face mask template
-

Instructions

First get the elastic and place on the paper template and cut it to the length of the paper which is about 11 inches .

Then cut out your template along the black outline using the fabric scissors.

 Open the packet of the HEPA vacuum bag there are two actually of it inside which is capable of producing eight face masks. four face masks from each of the vacuum bag

Unfold one of the vacuum bag and expand the four sides of it by making incision to bring out the inside and your bag should be able to lay flat

as shown below

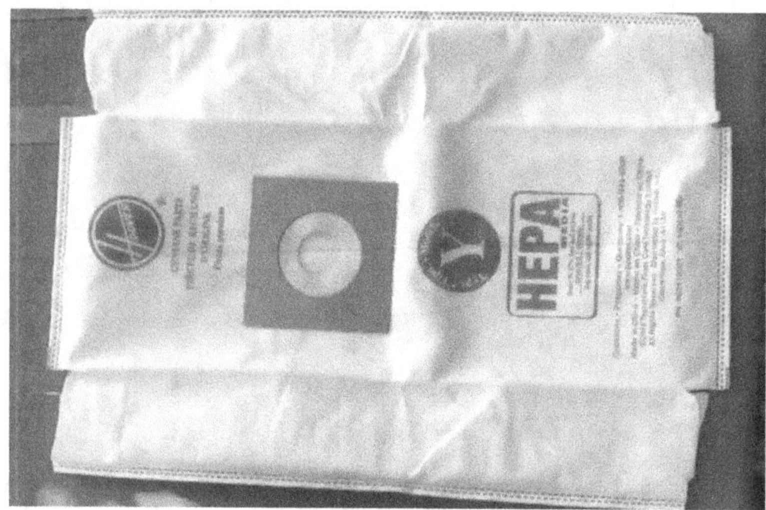

take your pattern and line it on the four

edges of the vacuum and make a trace. The reason
for using the edges is to get the mask to be sealed
enough to give the desired protection and do not
use pins to line the pattern and trace it because
we don't want holes on the mask in order to make
as safe as possible .

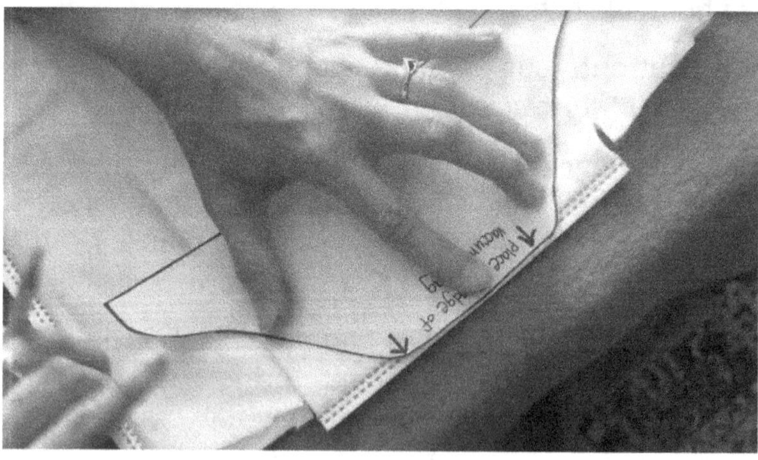

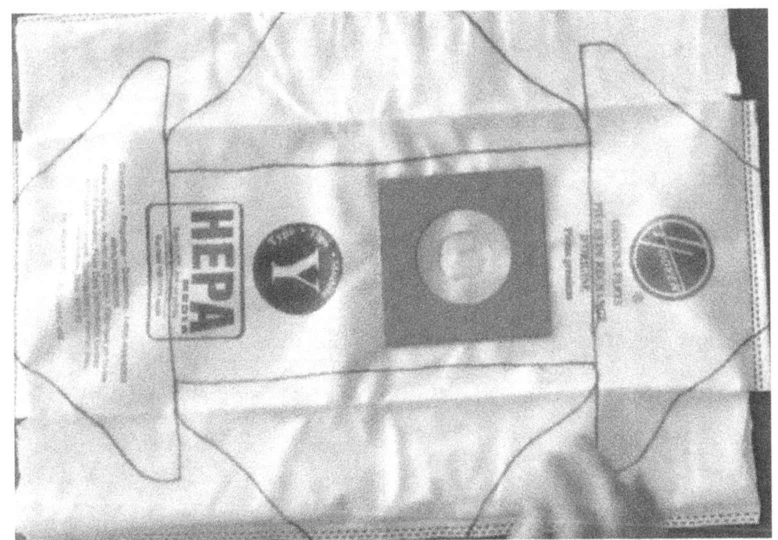

As you can see you can trace out four masks on one vacuum bag, you can do two regular face masks on the shorter ends and the smaller sized ones at the other two ends.

After tracing, you cut the masks out while cutting ensure that the bag is flat since we are not using pins to hold it down.

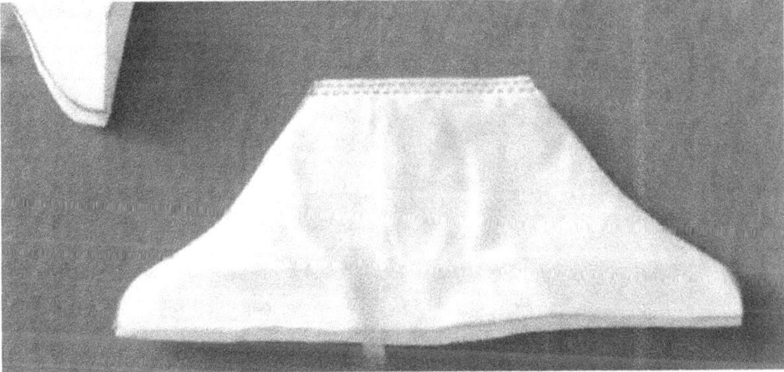

There is a part of the vacuum that is not part of the filter, so we cut it out, so you open the mask and cut out the nylon part

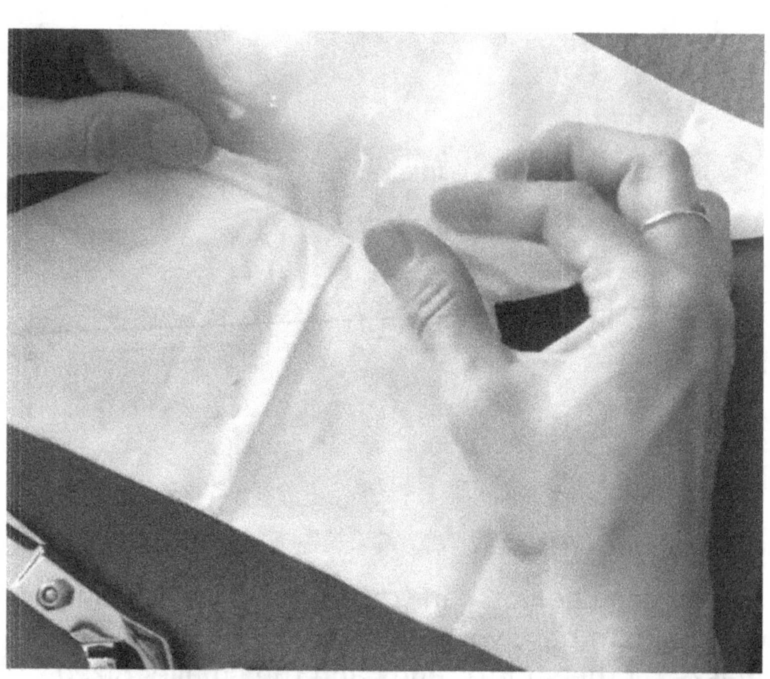

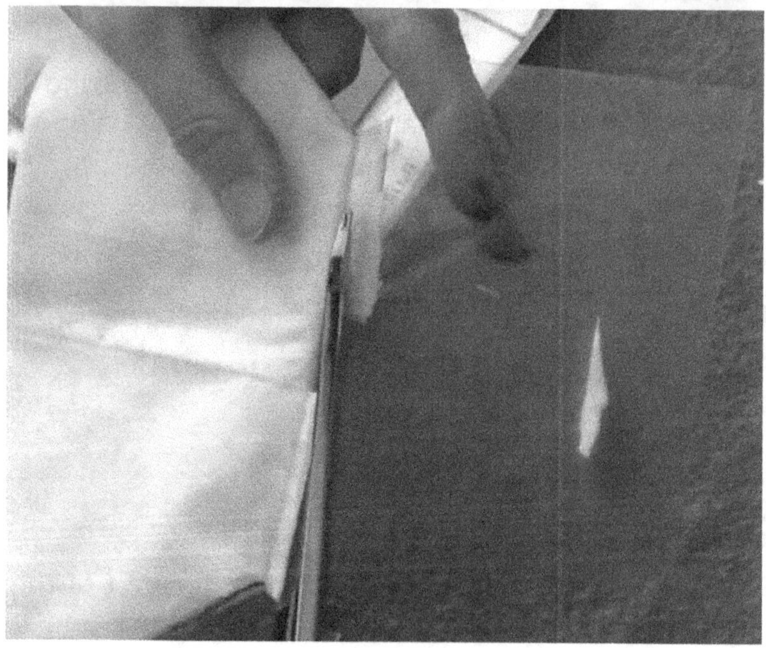

The next step is to insert the pipe cleaner into the face mask so that it will give weight to hold onto the nose when worn, take a pipe cleaner and fold into two or half

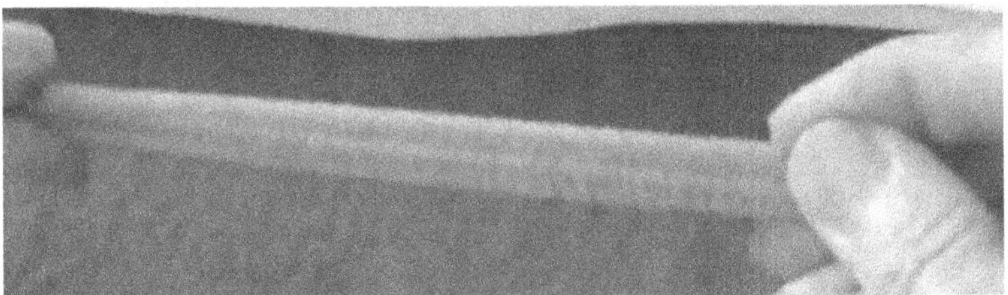

Then open the top layer of the mask which reveals a piece of plastic

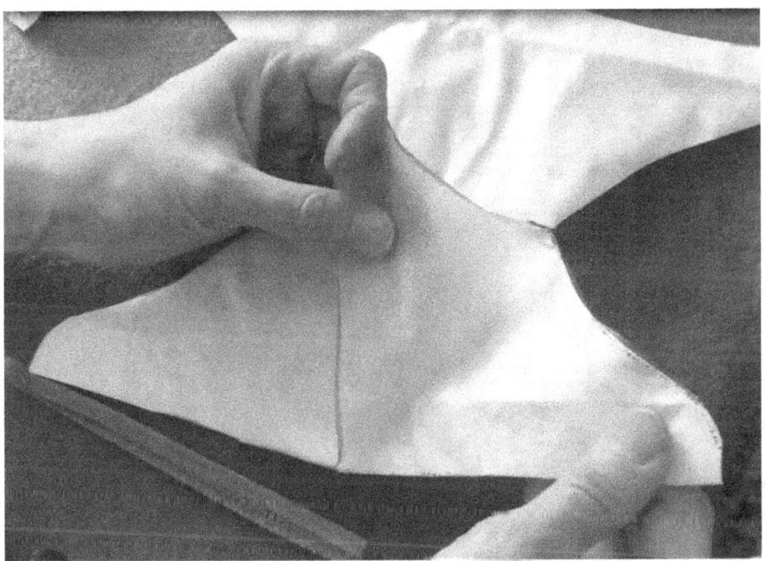

Place the folded pipe cleaner on it. place as shown below so as to have enough room to sew it up

Then smear the pipe cleaner with the glue and place it as shown below

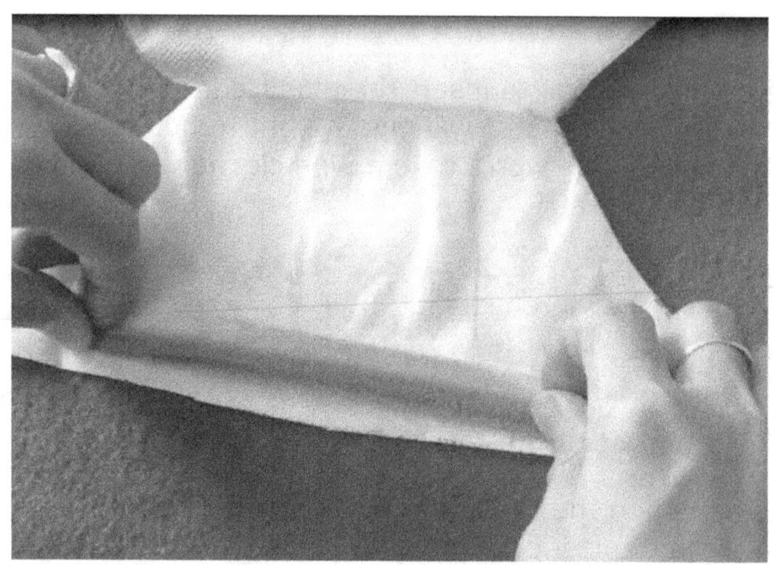

Press it down and cover back the top layer

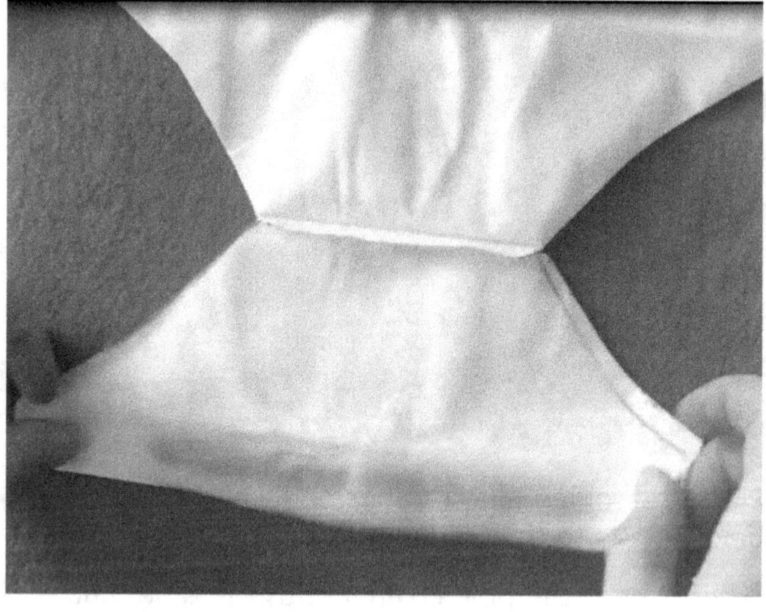

but make sure it doesn't gum the top layer also, so
you may need to open it again to ensure that the
gum didn't get to it   then cover it back again

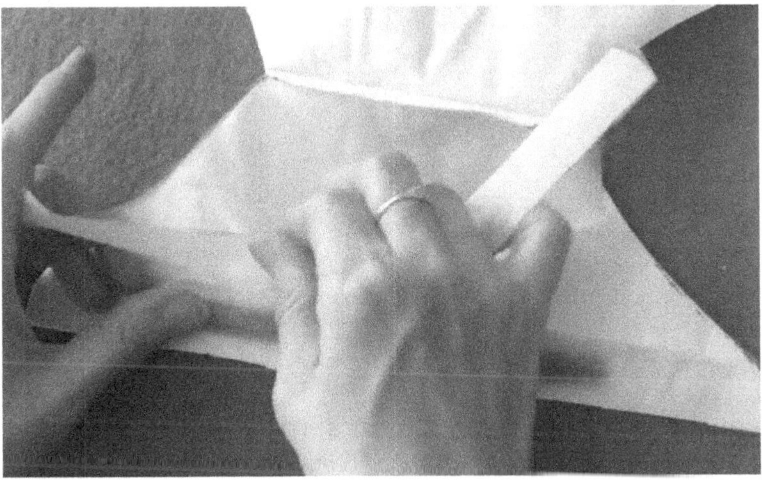

Then flip the mask over and place the elastic band
on it and sew the two sides of it to hold them to
the mask

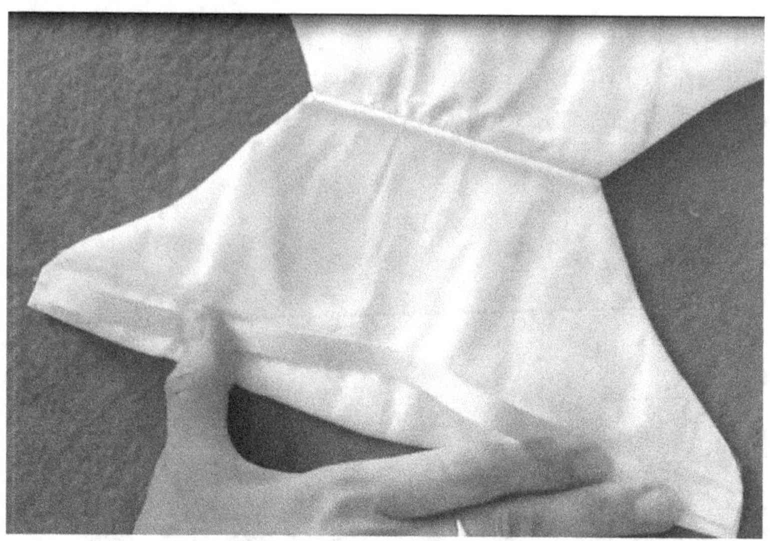

You are also going to do the same thing to the other side of the mask

Sew the pipe cleaner area firs and the two sides where the elastic bands are placed, use sewing machine to avoid puncturing the mask , but if you will be careful enough or don't have sewing machine then use needle and thread to sew it up carefully

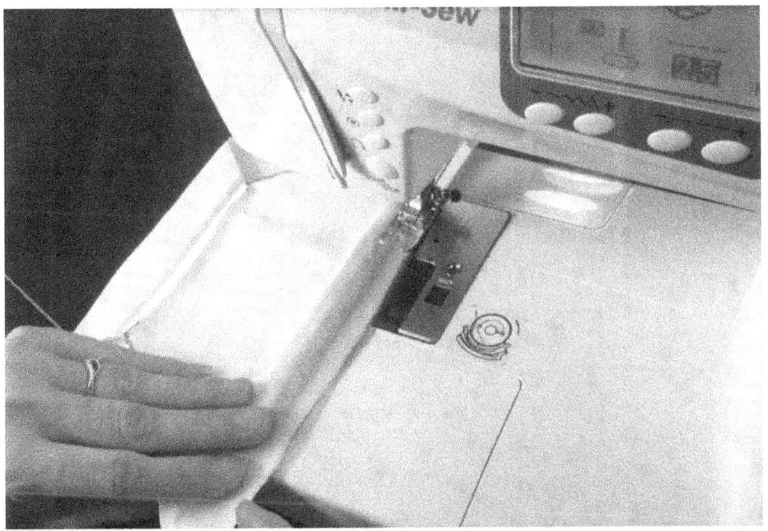

While sewing, you can always stop to reposition the mask fabric.

 Once you are done with sewing the pipe cleaner area and the four edges of the elastic band.

 The next thing is to sew along these edges as indicated by the red marker in the image below

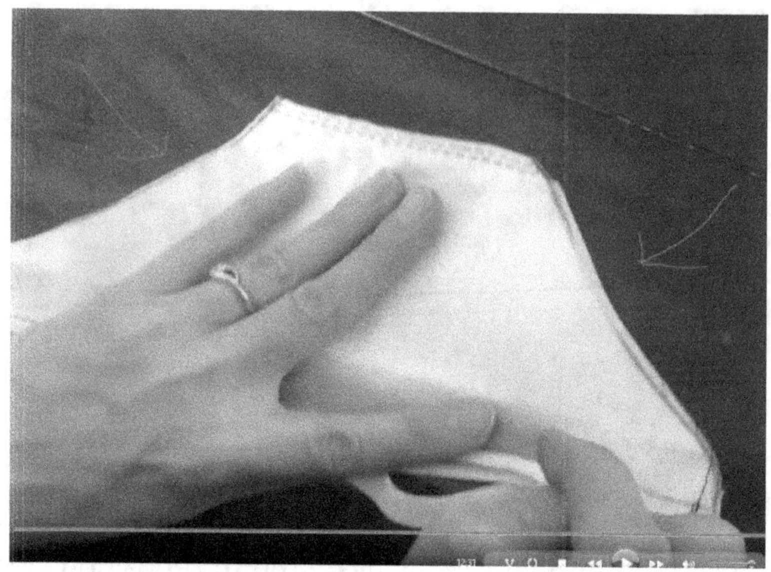

flip it and then sew a little bit closer on the inside
as indicated below

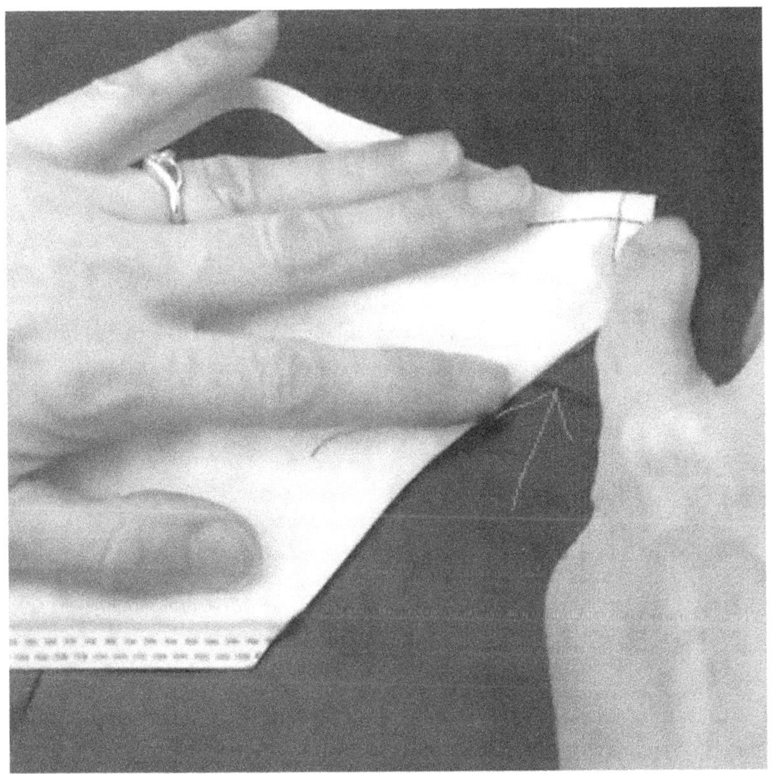

then trim off the excess thread and there you have your mask.

Repeat the same process for the remaining cut out patterns to get your face mask

Easy to do Face mask No sewing with Filter According to CDC recommendation

Materials

- 20 X 20-inch square of quilting material or hemp or extra-large T-Shirt- 100 cotton
- Two pieces of elastic band 6 inch each (or rubber bands or string, cloth strips, or 2 hair ties)
- Coffee Filter
- A pair of Scissor
- Pencil and ruler

Instructions

If you are using a T-Shirt, use a ruler and pencil and draw lines to measure out the 20 x 20-inch square, cut the edges off to get the measured 20 x 20-inch size.

Then use your scissor to cut on the two folded sides in between the two layers.

Take one piece the two squared fabric.

Fold the cloth by bringing the two edges in the midlle

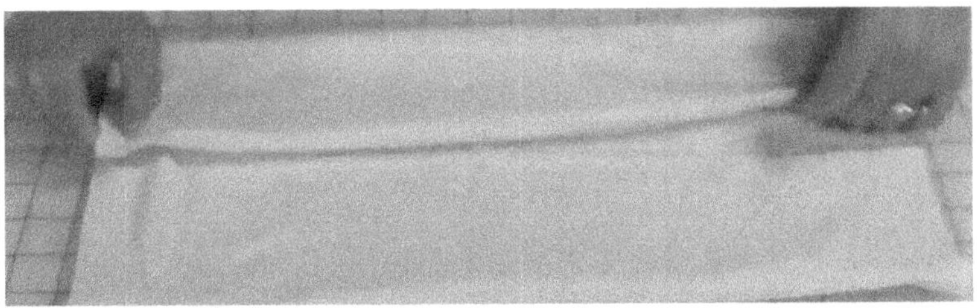

Then fold the coffee filter in half and insert it at the center of the folded fabric

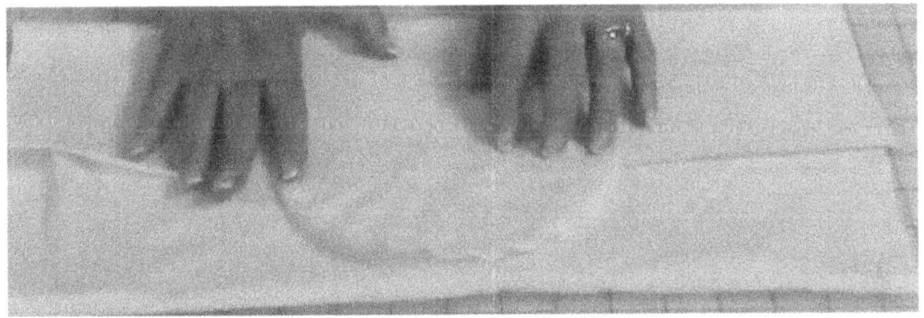

Then fold the fabric in half again and take your two hair ties or rubber bands and insert it through the end of the fabric do same for the both ends

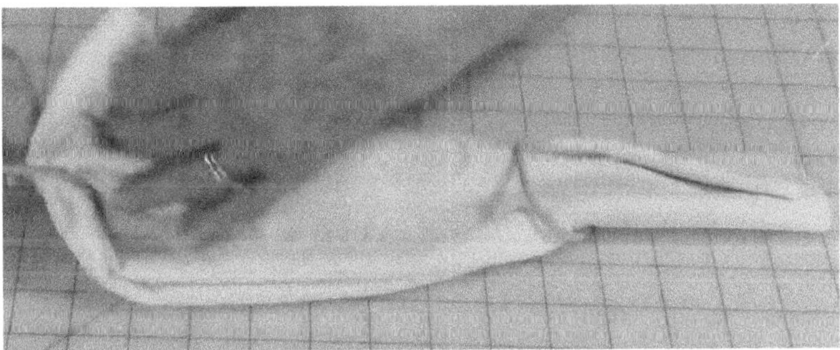

Then open the center and insert the two ends
underneath it fold the ends towards the middle

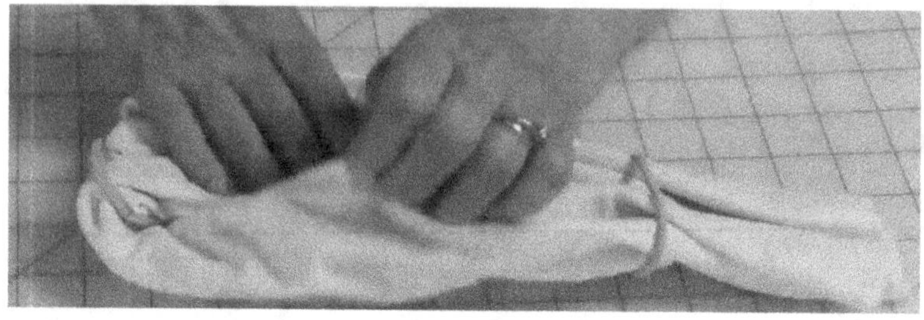

When you wear it should be like this

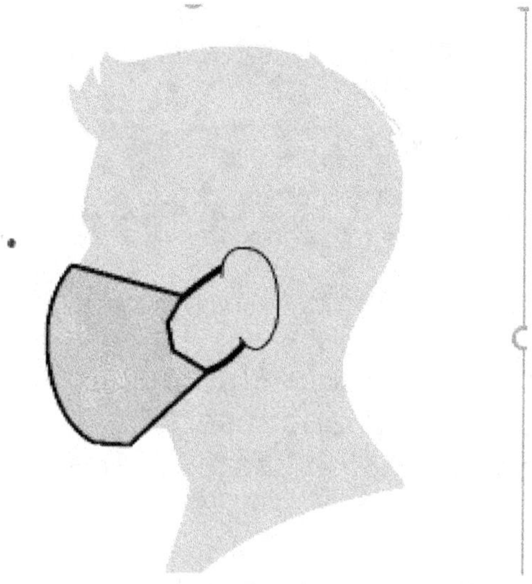

Disposable Face mask with paper Towel and panty liner as an effective filter

Materials

- A paper towels
- Two rubber bands
- Panty Liner
- A pair of Scissor
- Stapler

The reason for using magnetic panty liner is that it has a layer that is magnetic, anion and far infrared that effectively restricts the growth and survival of bacteria and viruses. It has a breathable premium cotton surface that is soft and comfortable, eliminate moisture and heat fast, keeping you fresh and soft air laid paper that enhances softness and freshness So, for a make shift face mask it should offer the same level of protection,

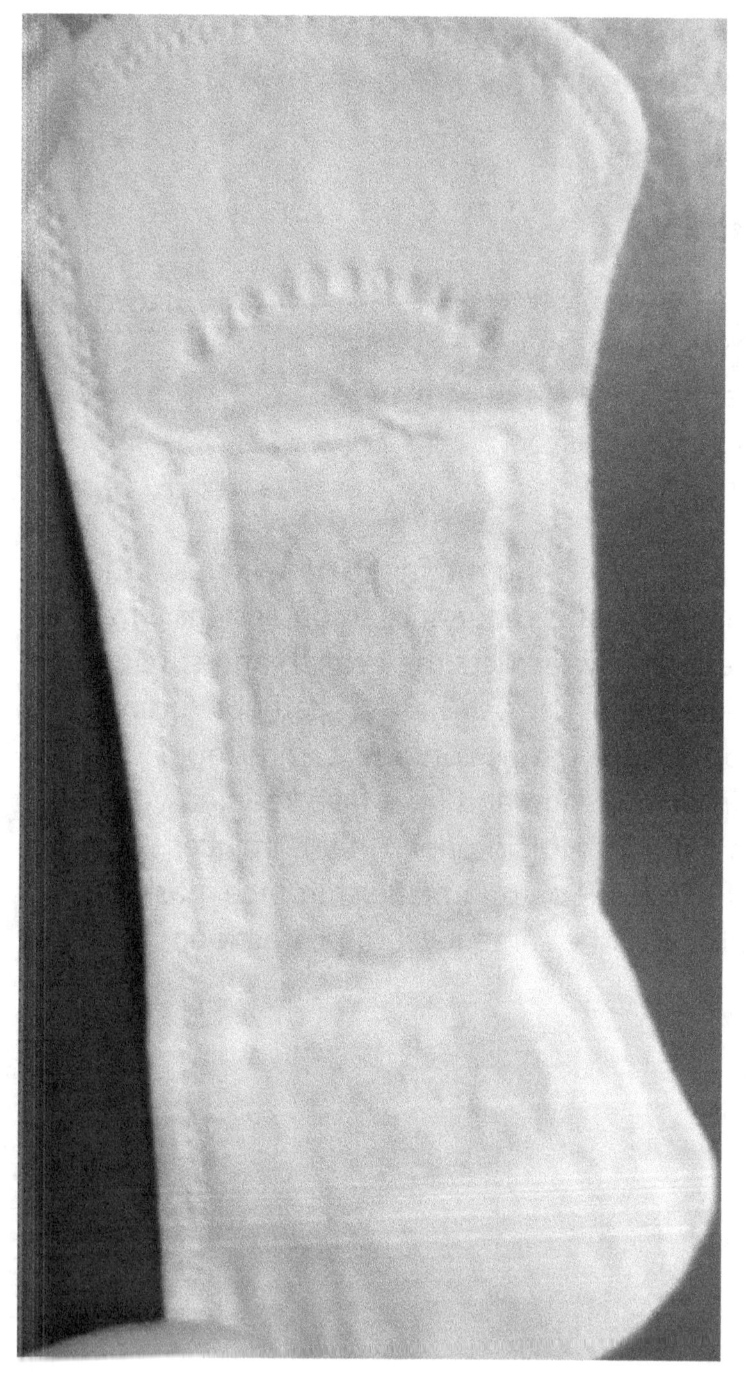

Instructions

 Lay the paper towel down and fold back and front like this

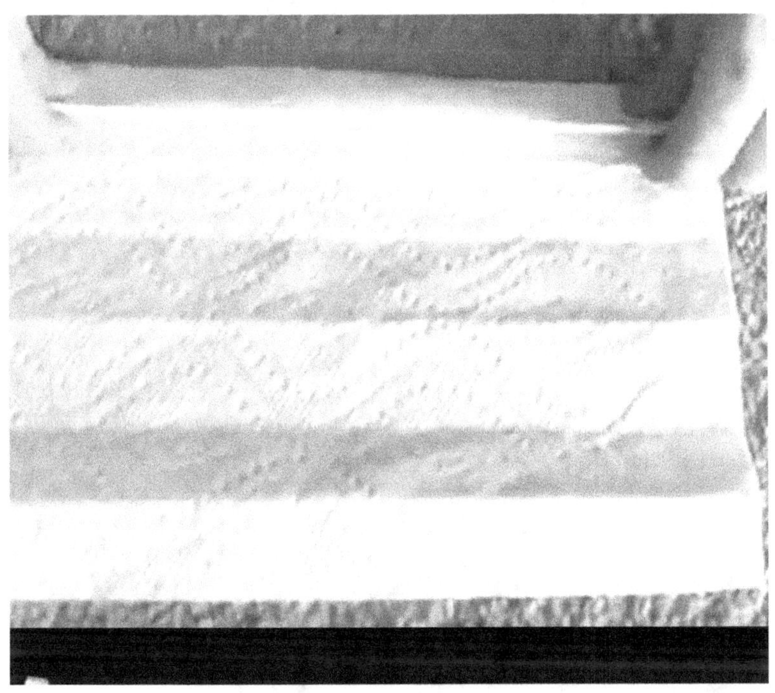

Until you have folded like this

Then take a rubber band and press in about
half inch from the end and fold it over on top of
the rubber band do same on the other end

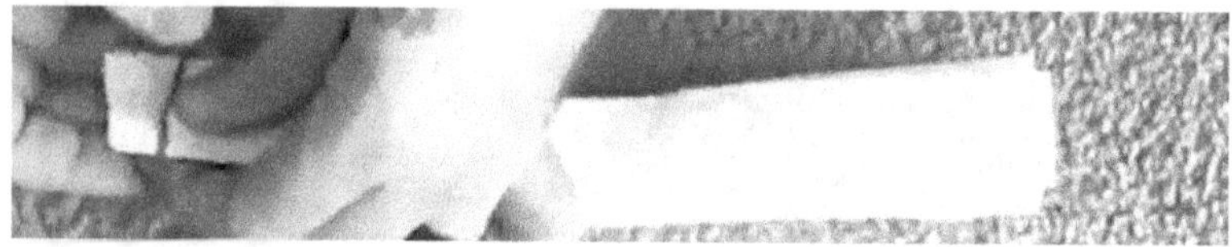

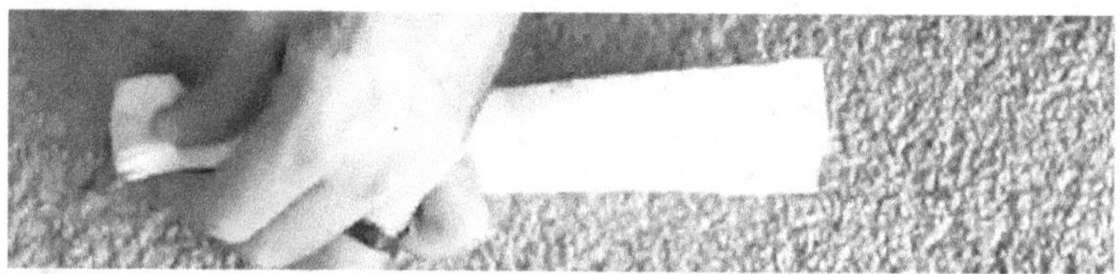

Then using a stapler, staple the folded edges

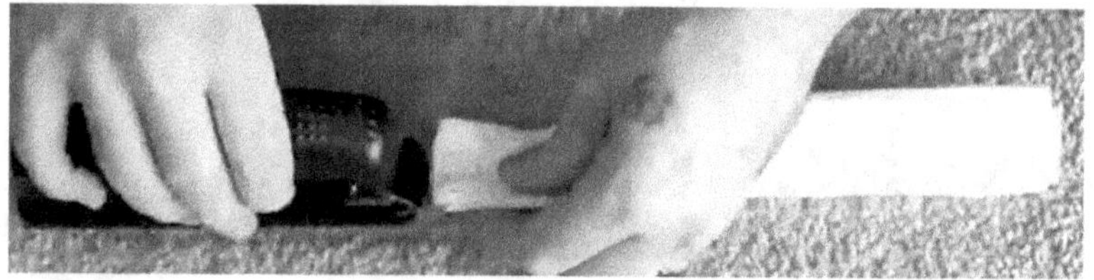

After that you should have something like this

Then get a pant liner open the nylon and peel off
the strip to reveal the adhesive part then insert the
panty liner   at the center of the mask with the
adhesive part gumming to the mask   then you are
good to go. you can wear your mask remember
that it is not reusable

Three minutes T-shirt Face Mask without Elastic (no sewing Required)

Materials

- T-shirt
- Scissors

Instruction

1.

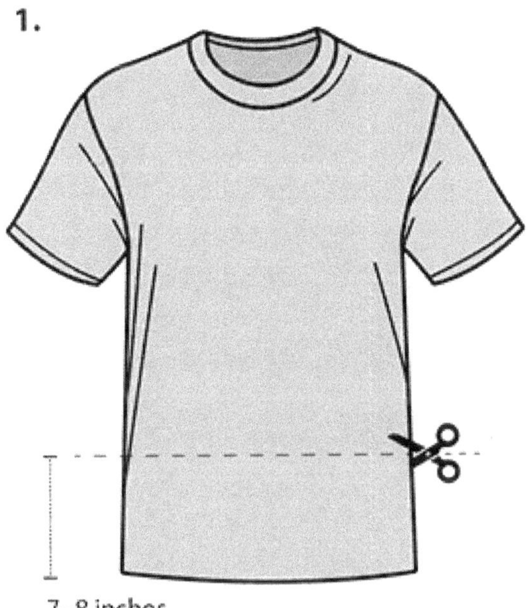

2.

6–7 inches
cut out
cut tie strings

3.

Tie strings
around neck,
then over top
of head.

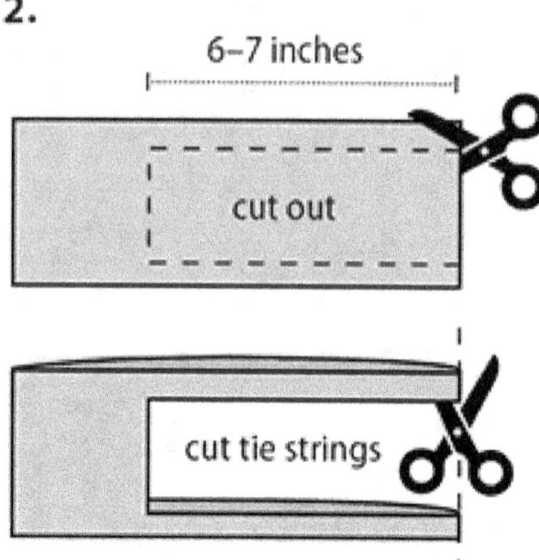

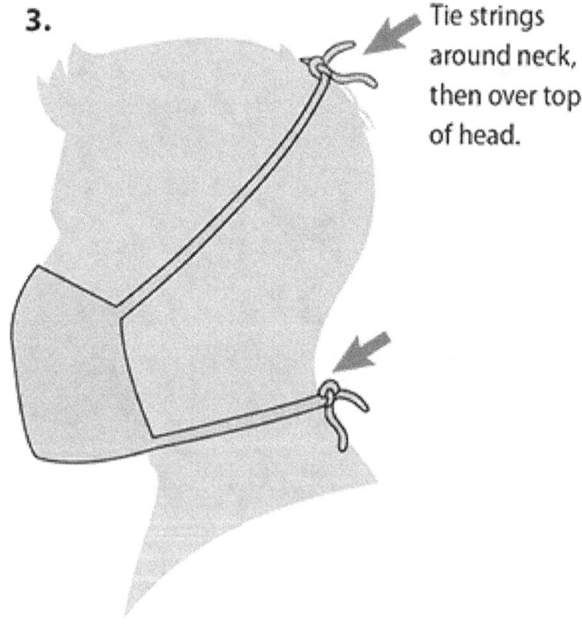

Bandana Face Mask without Elastic (no sewing method)

Materials

- Bandana (or square cotton cloth of 20"x20")
- Rubber bands (or hair ties)
- Scissors

Instruction

1. 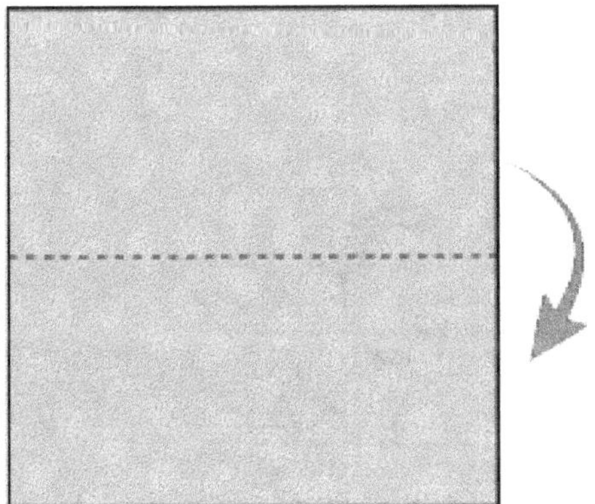

Fold bandana in half.

2.

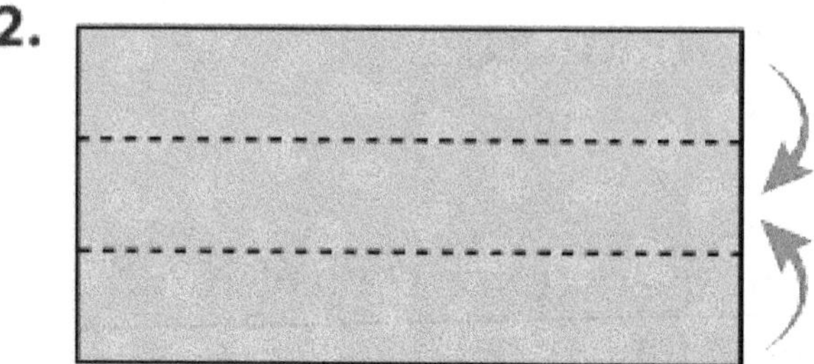

Fold top down. Fold bottom up.

3.

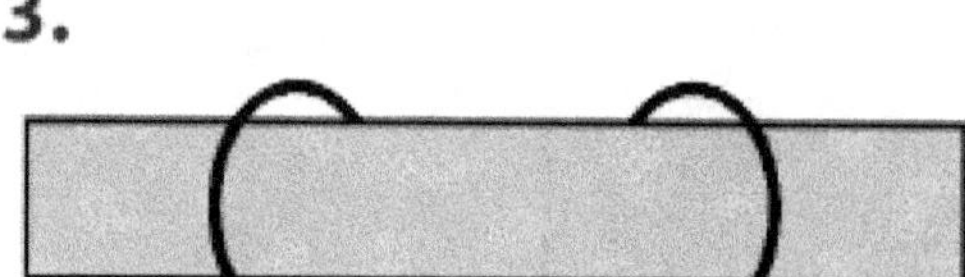

Place rubber bands or hair ties
about 6 inches apart.

4.

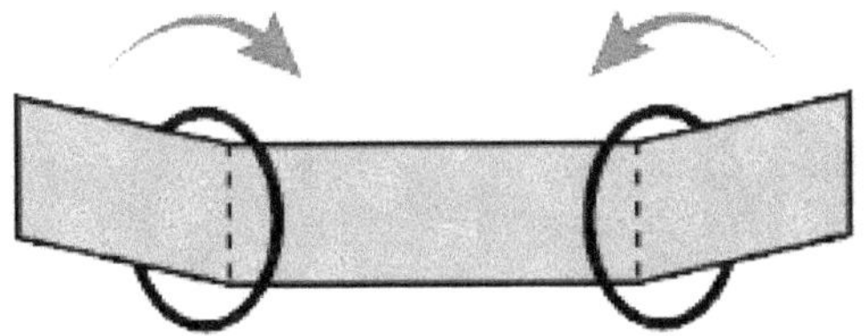

Fold side to the middle and tuck.

5.

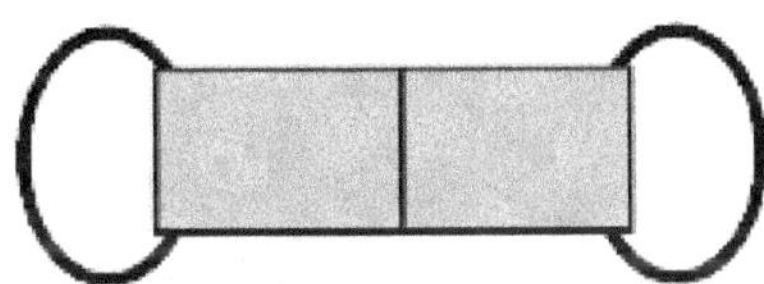

6.

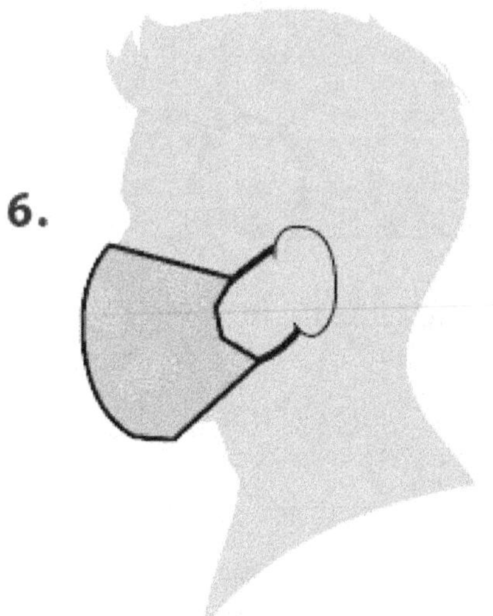

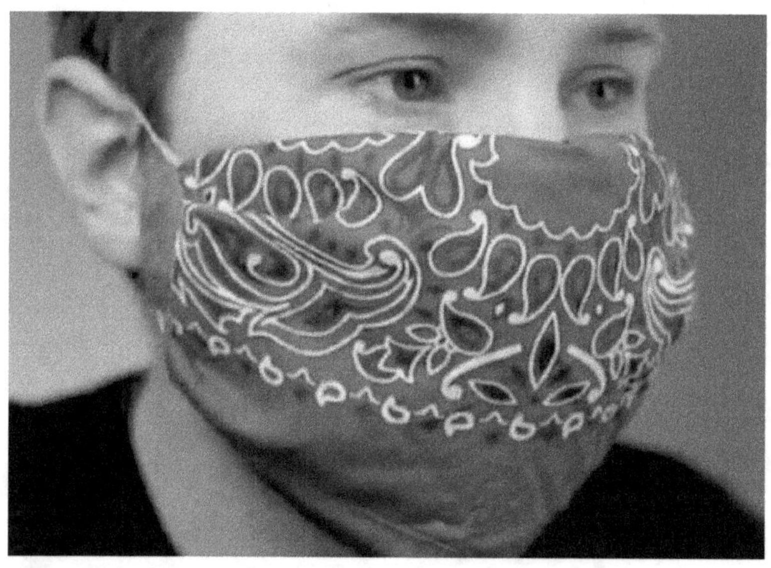

Reusable washable Face mask with a filter pocket such that you can always replace the filter: the mask is comfortable to wear without Ear sore

Materials

- Sewing pins or clips
- Rotary cutter or a pair of scissors
- seven-inch piece of plastic-coated gardening wire
- 60" inch piece of synthetic clothesline (3/16" diameter)
- 100 % cotton fabric that is washed and dried

Instructions

Take your fabric and cut three pieces of your fabric 10-inch-wide and 8 inches high you will use one piece for your exterior and the other two fabrics for your interior, this will be the pieces that will have the filter in them

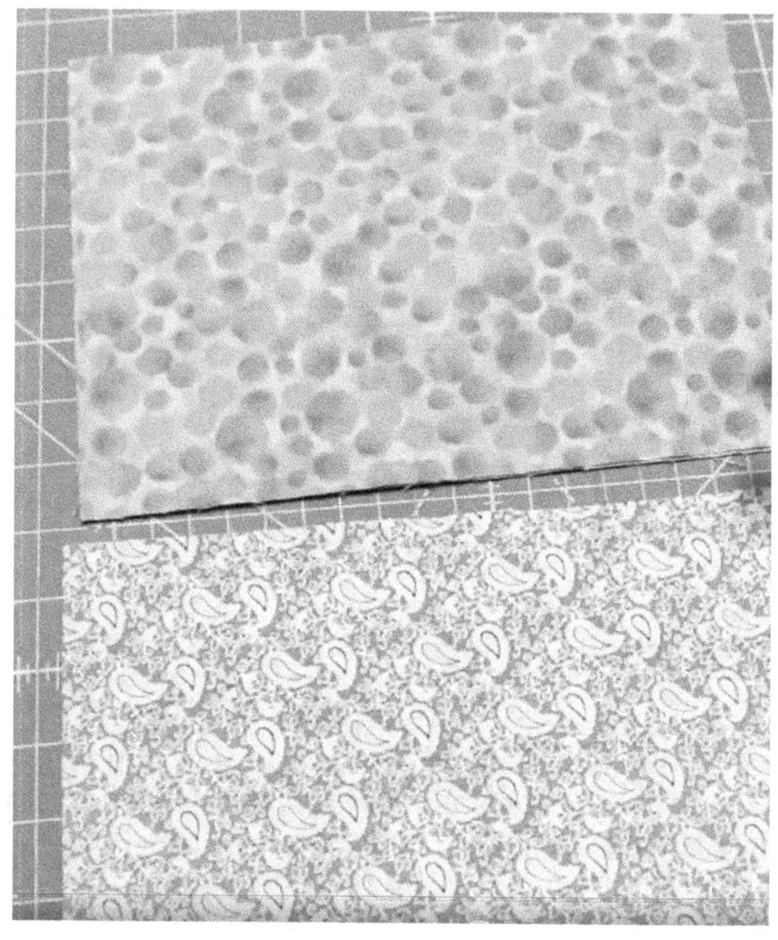

Take the two interios pieces and lay them
right sides together

Then fold in half length wise and gently press
down to make a crease

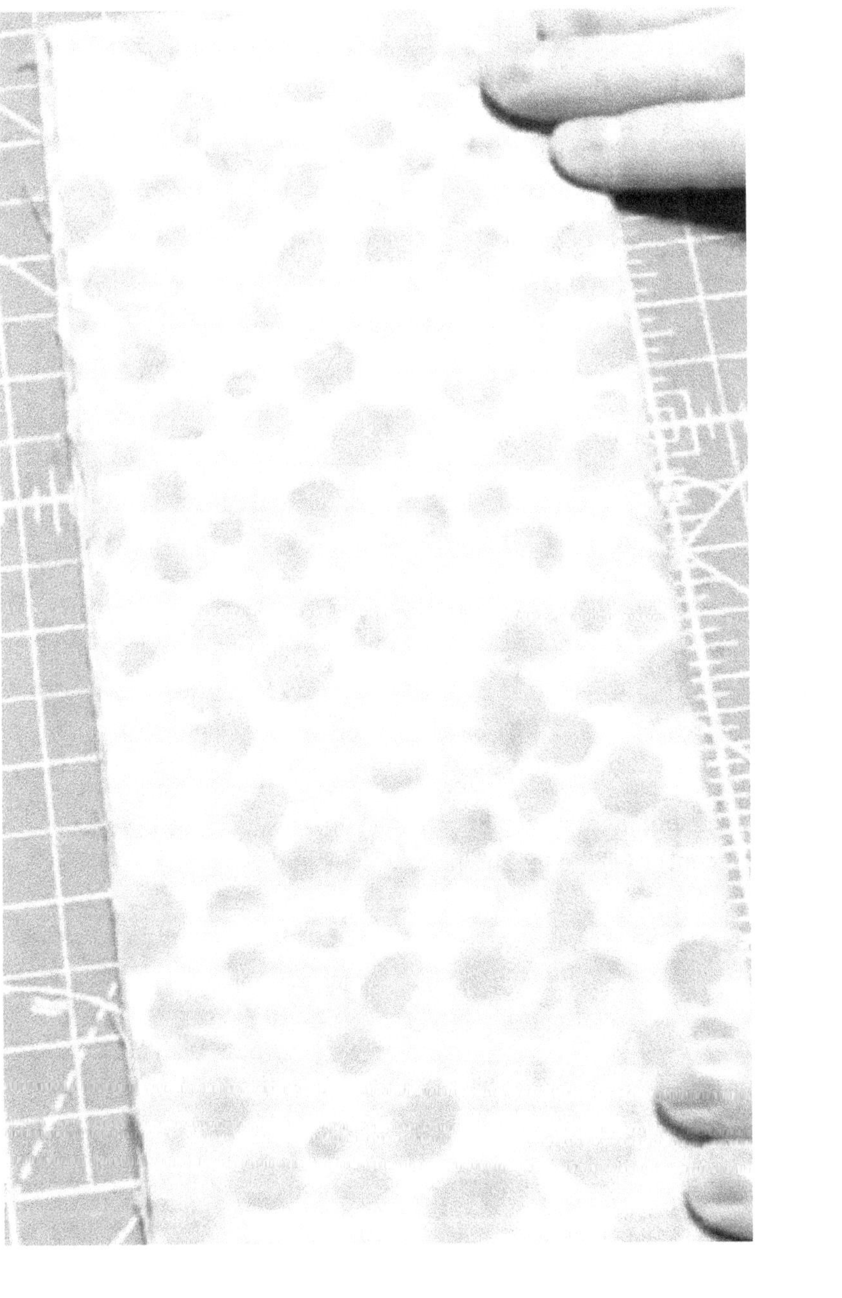

Open it back and Lay a ruler on the crease you just made

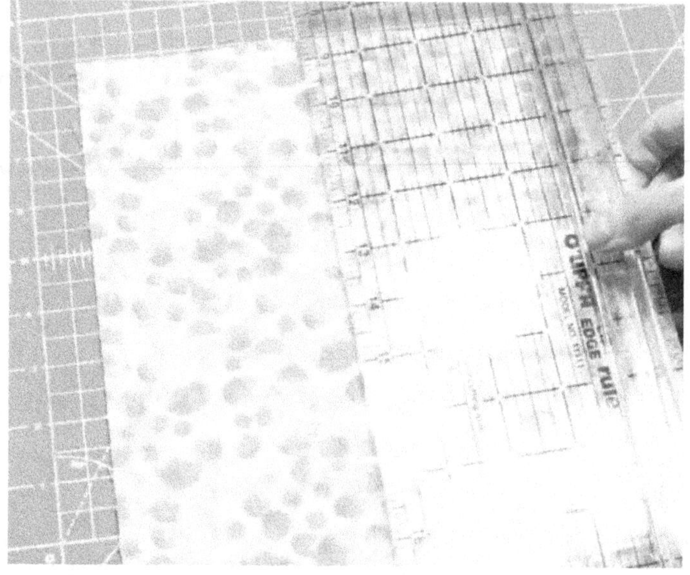

Take a pen and draw a 3 inch line from each side, the space in the center will be for the filter.

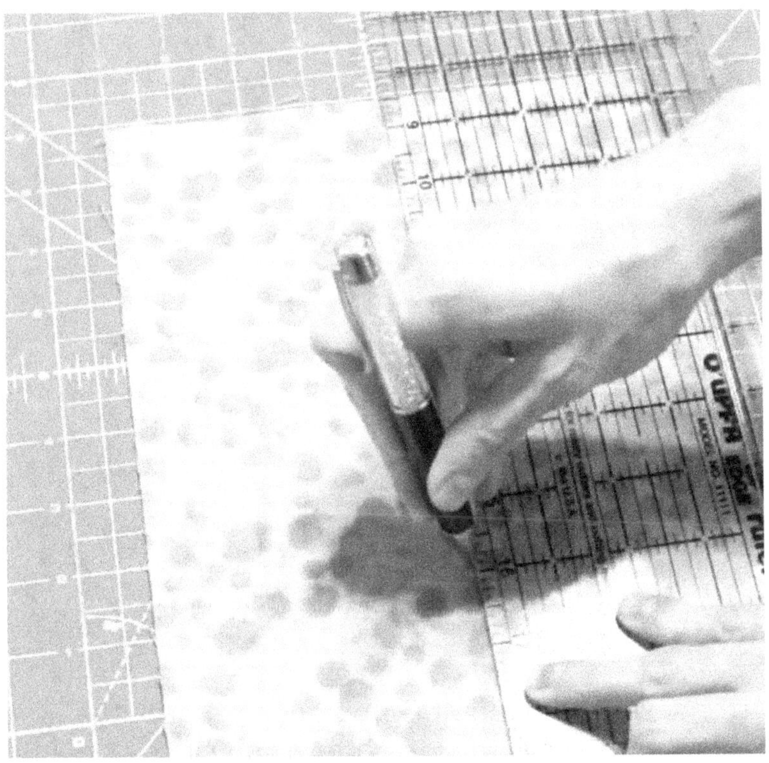

Sew down the lines you just made. Be sure and backstitch at the beginning and end of each line as indicated by the red marker

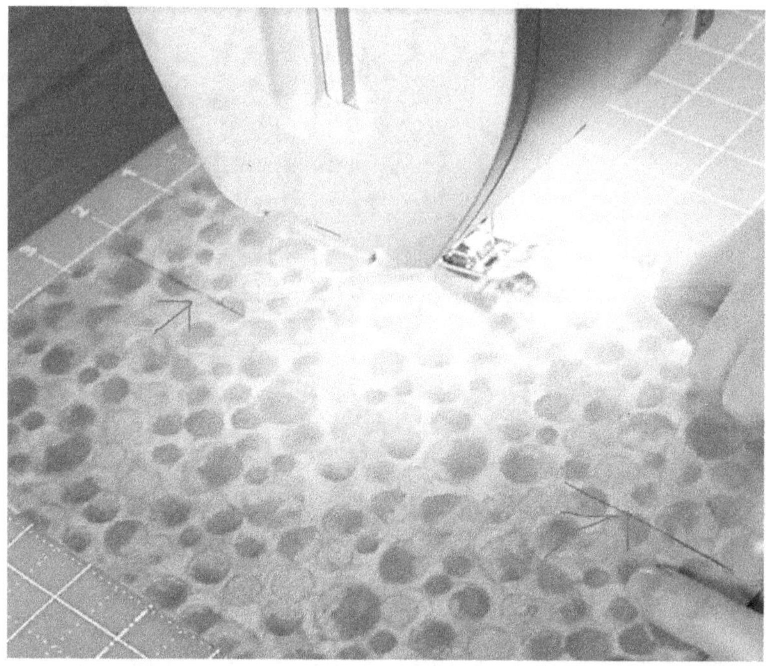

After sewing Fold up one long edge to meet the other and press with iron. The wrong sides of the fabric should be together

Flip the fabric over and repeat. When press open, you will have an opening in the center for the filter

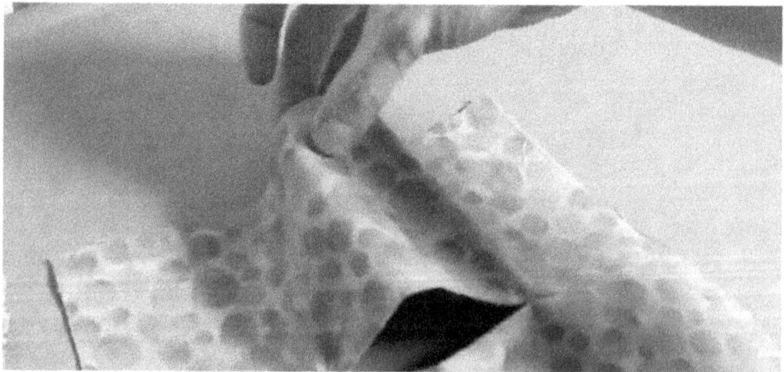

Also you can topstitch down the side of the seam.
this will help to reinforce the filter pocket

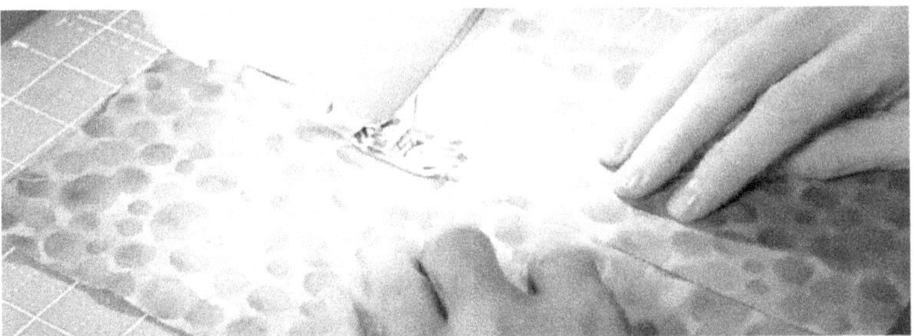

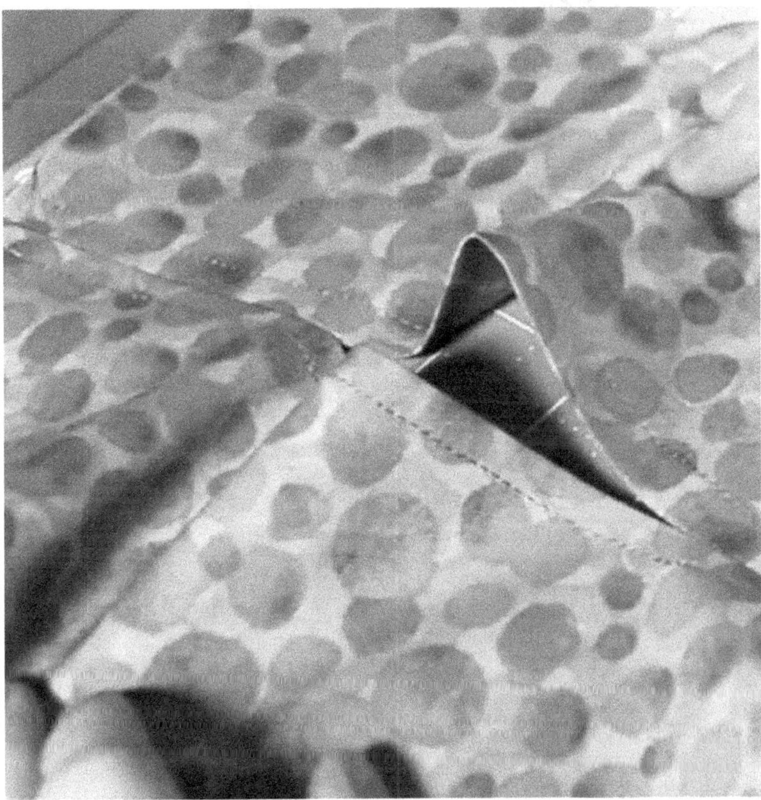

Now take the exterior piece of your mask and lay it
facing up and take your filter pocket and lay it on
top of the exterior fabric

Then stitch the four sides of the joined fabrics.
After that take scissor and snip off the edges of the
fabric to ease the turning out

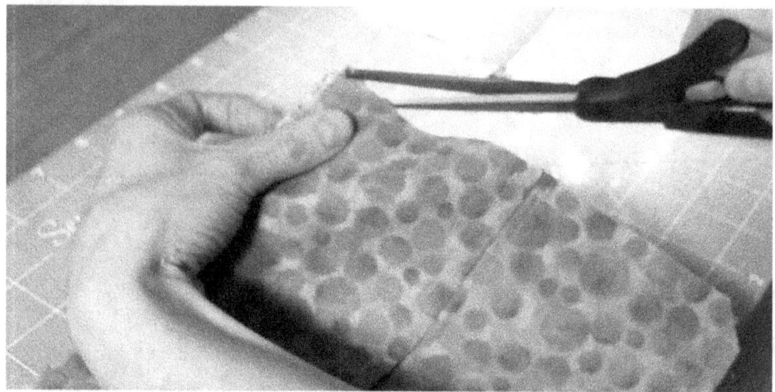

From the opening in the filter pocket turn the
mask inside out and carefully push out the four
corners of the fabric

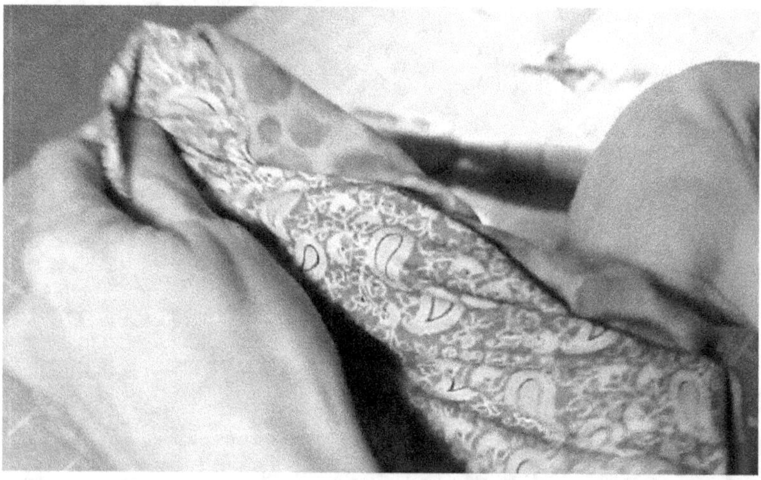

Press it with iron gently. After that place your mask
with the filter pocket facing up and fold up of the
ends the 8 inch side

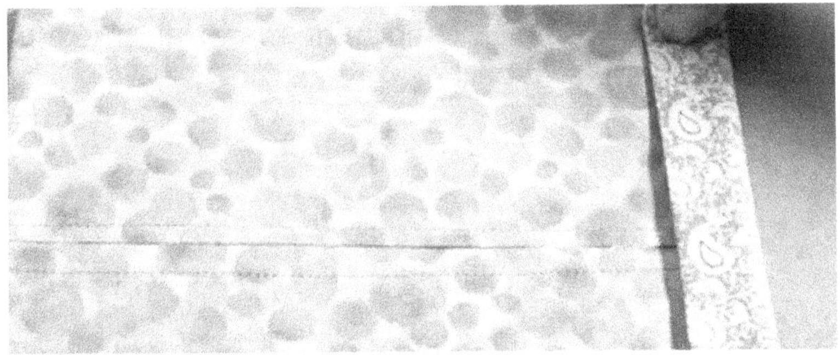

And give it a press

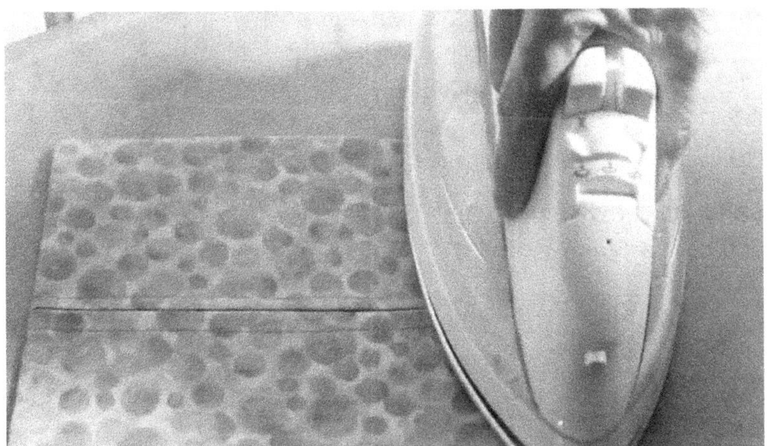

And do the same thing to the other side

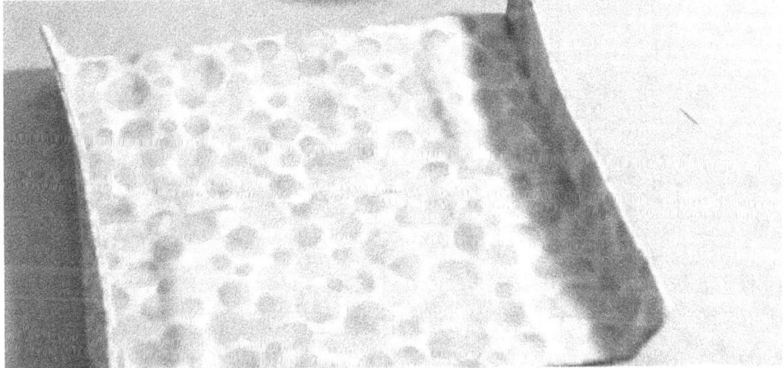

Now get the clothesline synthetic material make a knot at the two end of it

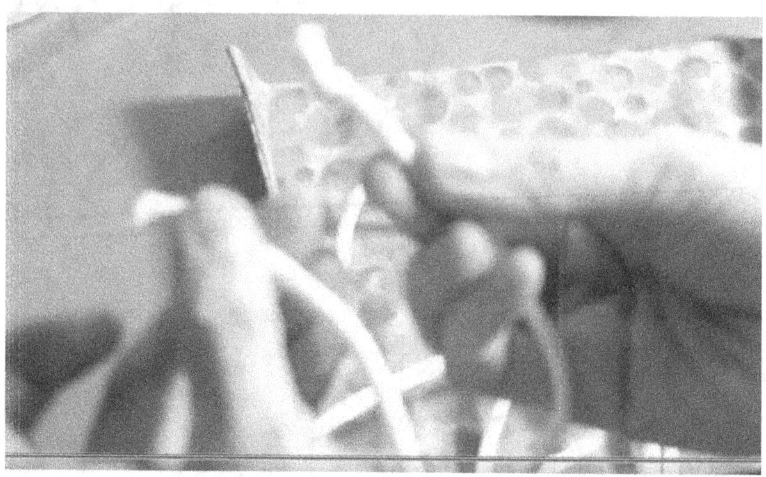

Lay the clothesline along the folded path of the mask to form a loop

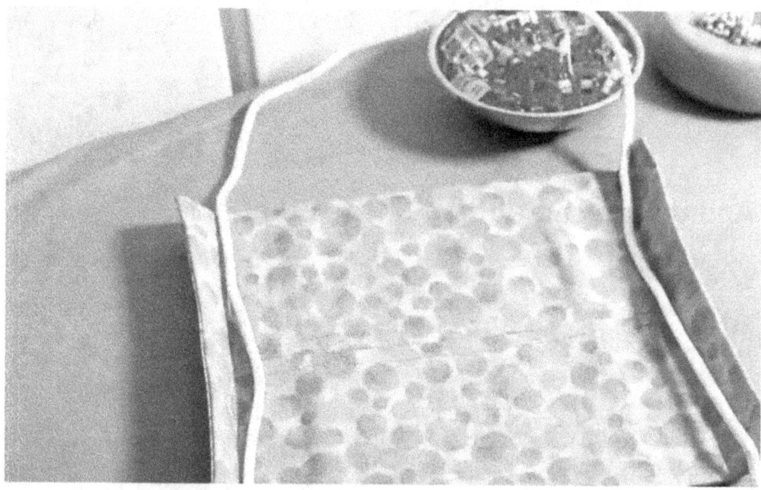

Then tuck in the edge of this folded part by folding it in a triangular way and fold the entire edge over the rope and clip the two ends to hold it down

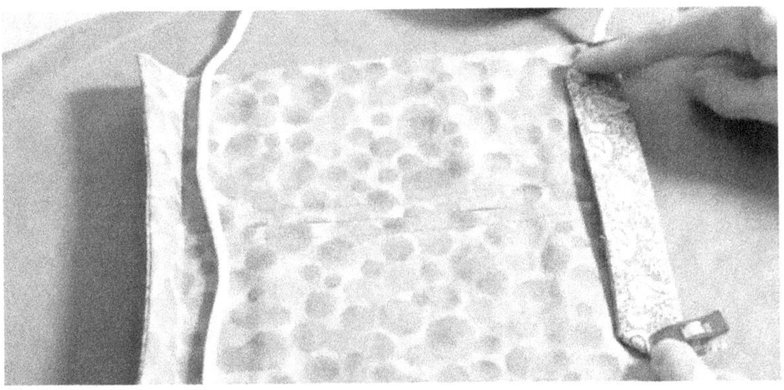

Do same for the other edge

You will sew from the top of the folded edge of the mask all the way down and ensure that you backstitch also do same for the two folded edges be careful not to sew through the clothesline cord

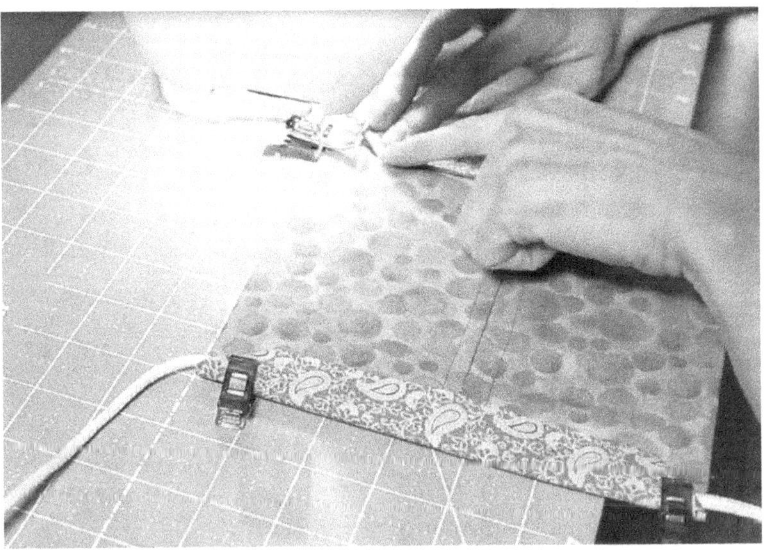

Get the seven-inch gardening wire and fold the edge one inch to itself to ensure that the sharp edges of the wire are not coming out to avoid poking you when you wear the mask   do same at

the other end of the wire . you ma y need plier to
clip the edges in

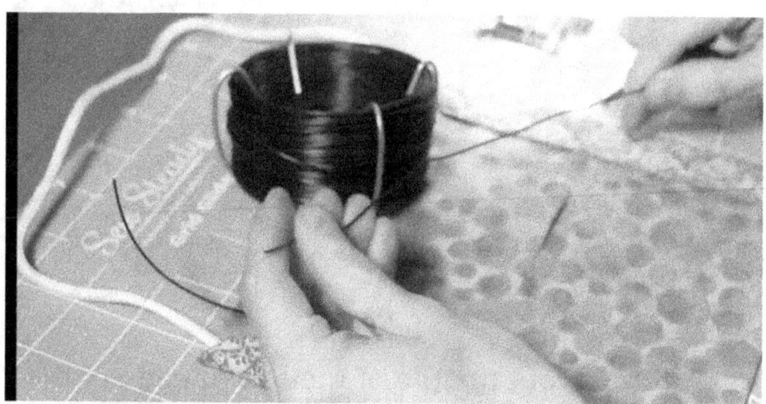

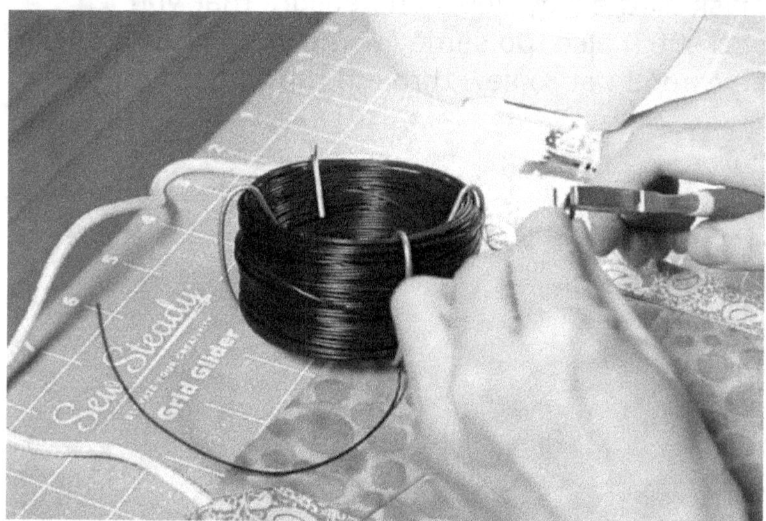

 Slide in to the top of the mask through the filter
pocket opening. the top of the mask is the place
where the knot of the clothesline that will go over
your head is seen. Slide the wire in and push it to
the edge an them sew from top to the bottom of it
to hold it in that position

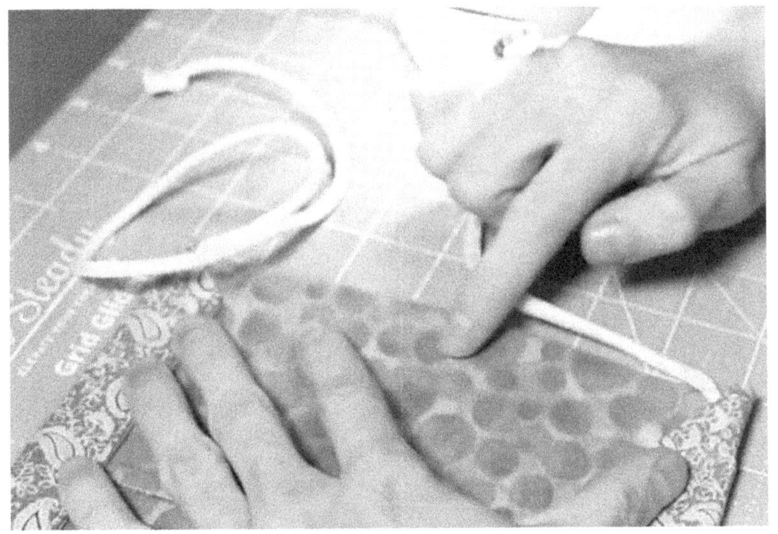

When sewing you have to be careful so than you don't sew over the wire and break your needle

After that your mask is ready for wear

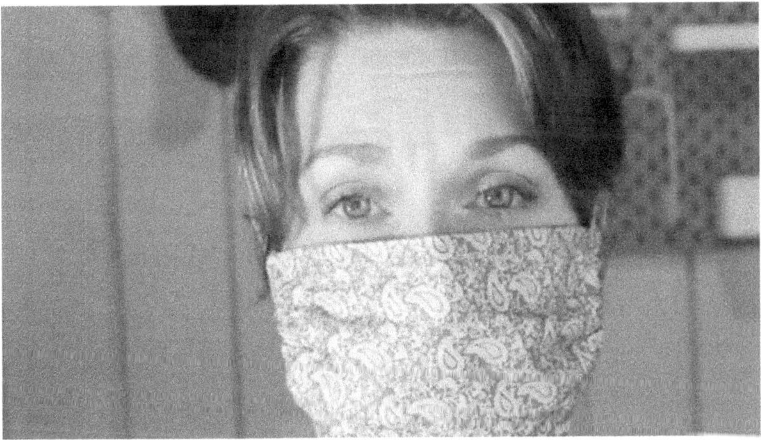

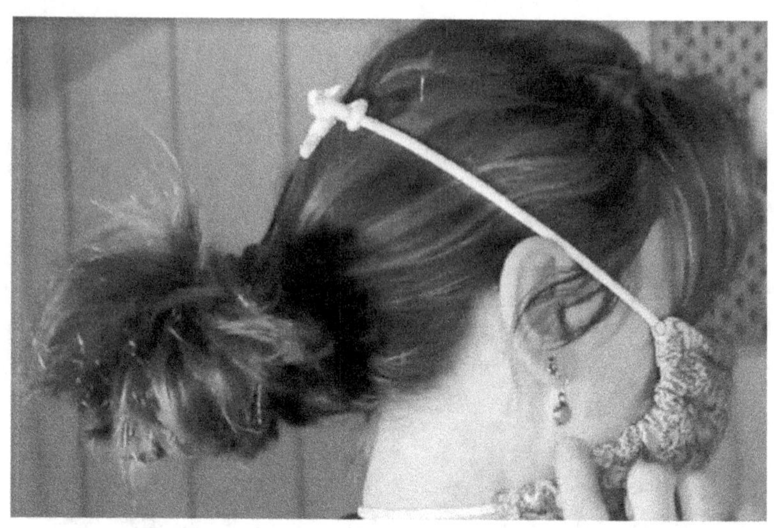

Oh remember that you can always replace the
Filter through the filter pocket

Adding a Fitted Nose to the Face Mask
Materials

- Sewing clips
- Ribbons
- Pipe Cleaner or gardening wire
- Needle and thread or sewing machine

Instructions

You add this fitted nose to already made face mask

First cut out the ribbon about two and half inches long

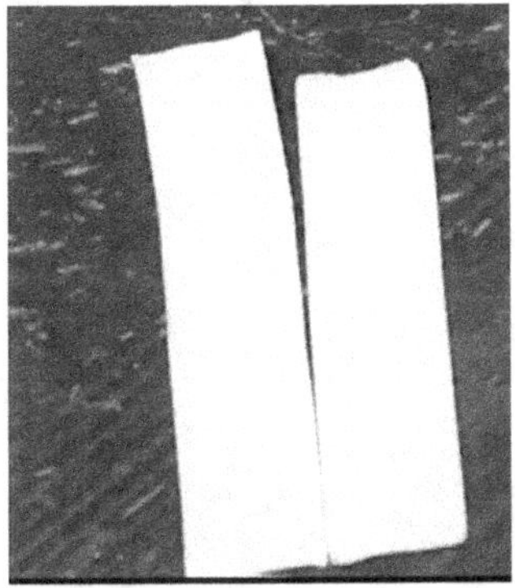

Then use the lighter to seal edges to avoid frayed ends

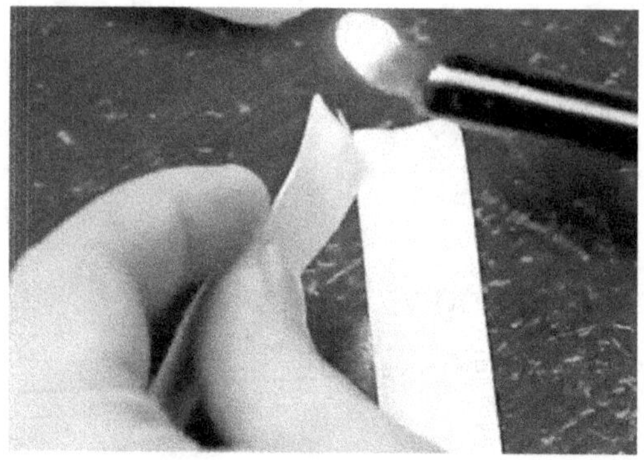

 Get your mask and fold it in half and position the ribbon at the top of the mask where the mask will be positioned on your nose and clip the ribbon in position

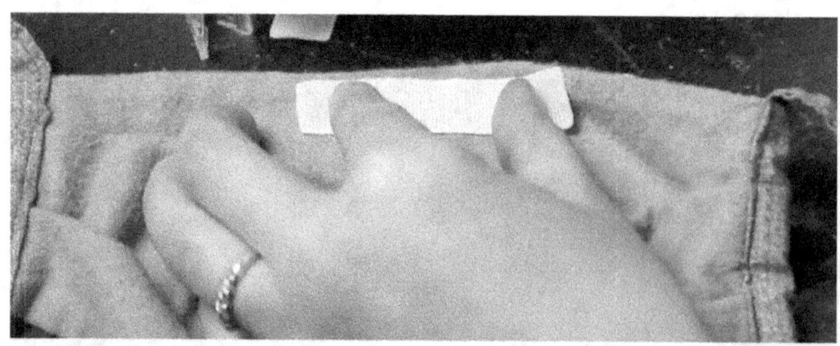

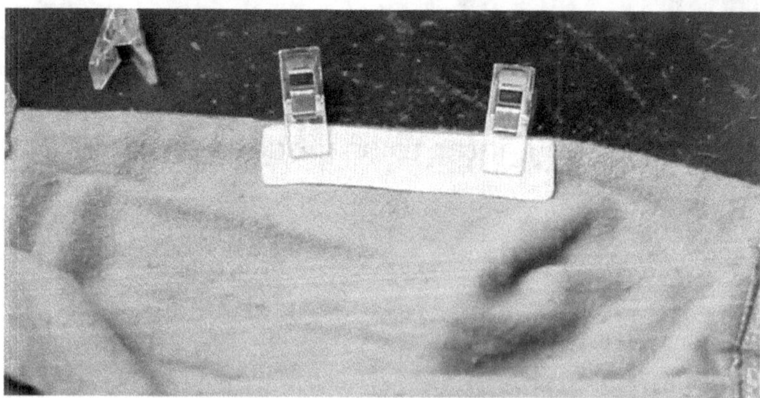

Then sew from all the edges of the ribbon except for the one indicated by the red marker because that is where you are going to insert the wire or the pipe cleaner to give it that nose fitting shape you can also use hand sewing to achieve this also

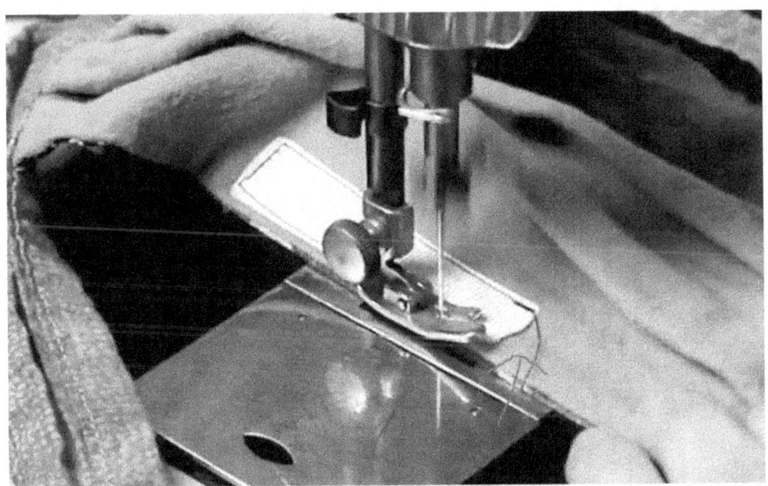

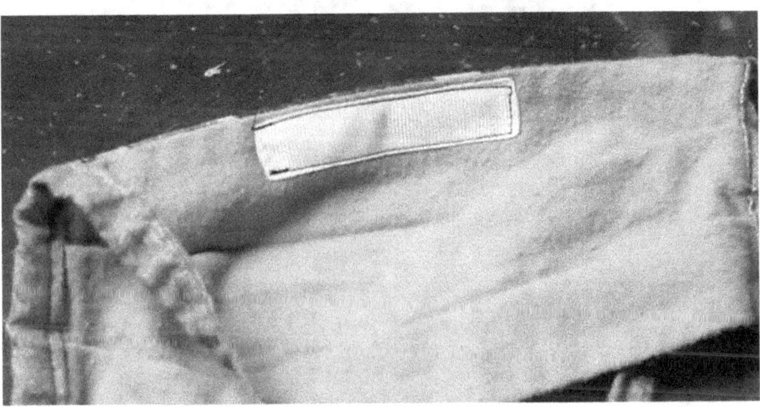

then get you pipe cleaner and fold into two and cut a size a little shorter than the ribbon length then fold the mouth so that they will

not be poking out and hold it together and
twist a little so that they hold tightly

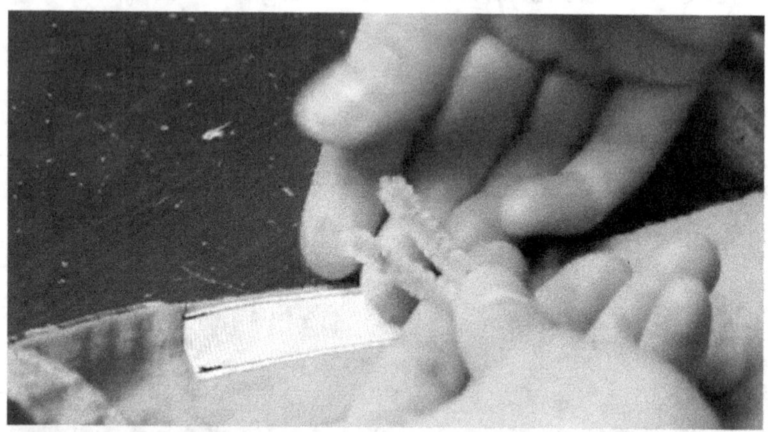

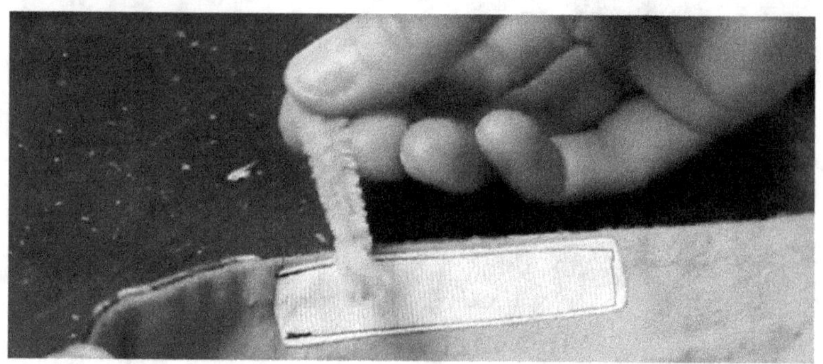

Then slip it in into the ribbon with the twist
end going in first

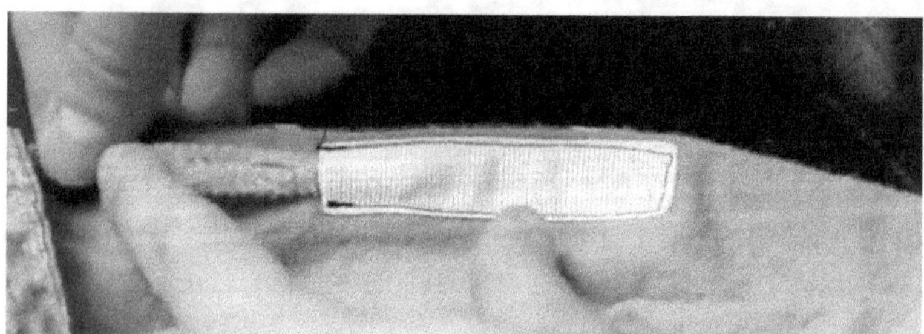

When you put on your mask simply bend the pipe cleaner so as to hug your nose and give that nose fitted shape

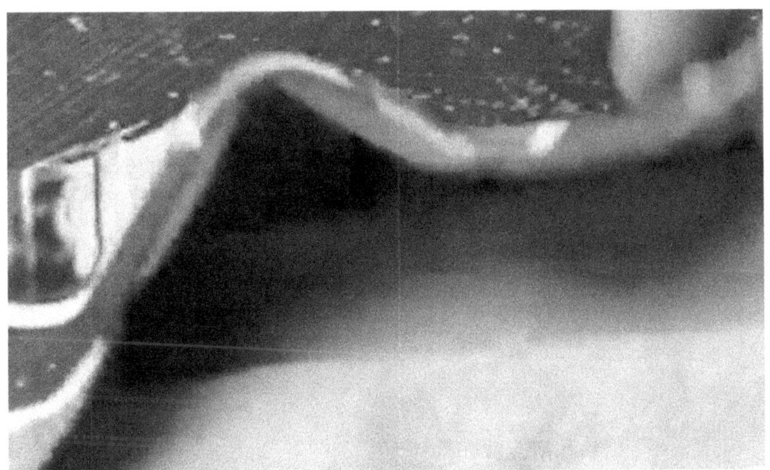

Remember to always take out the wire when you are about to wash your facemask

Making and Adding Ear savers or facemask adapters to your Face Mask

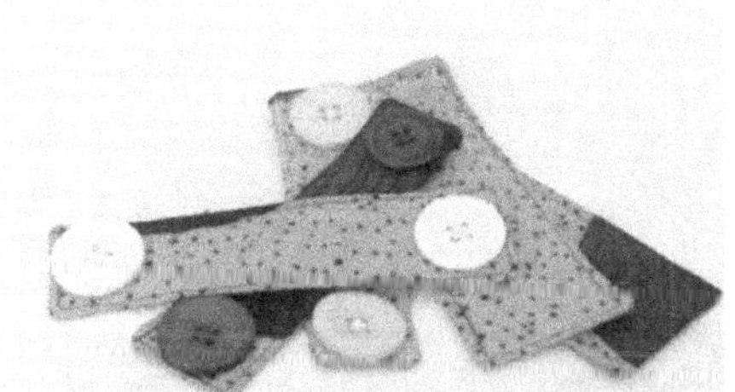

Materials

- Sewing needle and thread
- Two buttons size between ¾ and 1 inches

- Scrap fabrics
- Needle and thread or sewing machine
- Rotary cutters

Instructions

Cut out two pieces of cloth from your scrap material about 2 inches wide and 5.5 inches high of the fabric using your rotary cutter or scissor

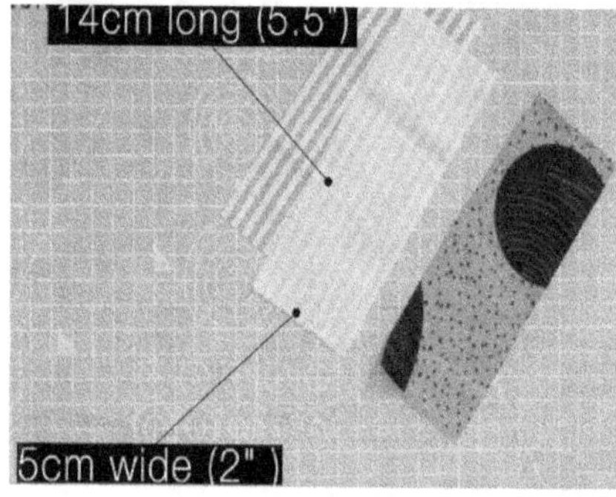

Sew all round the two fabrics leaving an opening of 2 inches

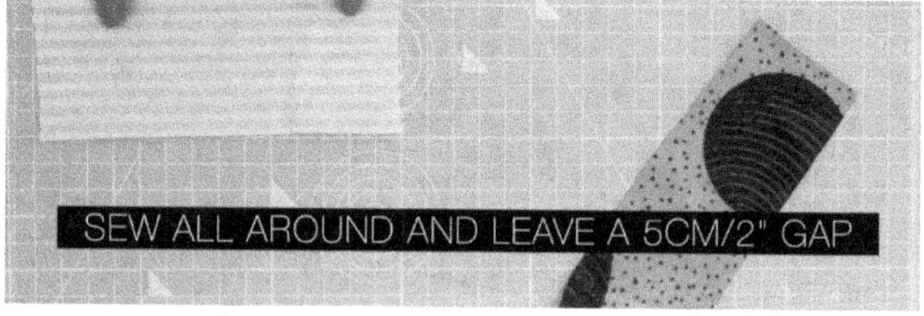

After sewing trim, the corners carefully and turn it inside out to reveal the opening

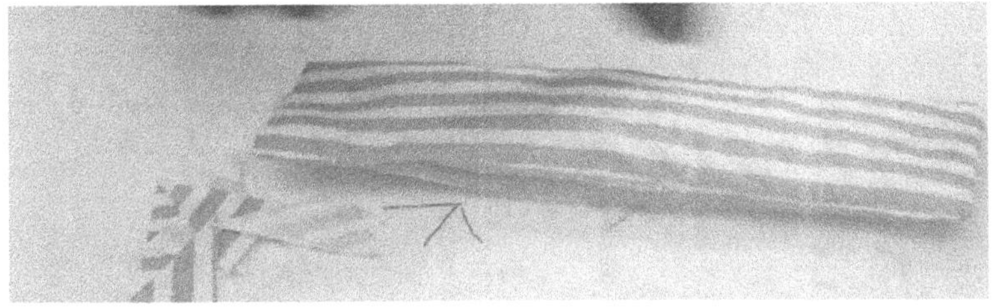

 Gently iron it and top stitch the four edges of the strip

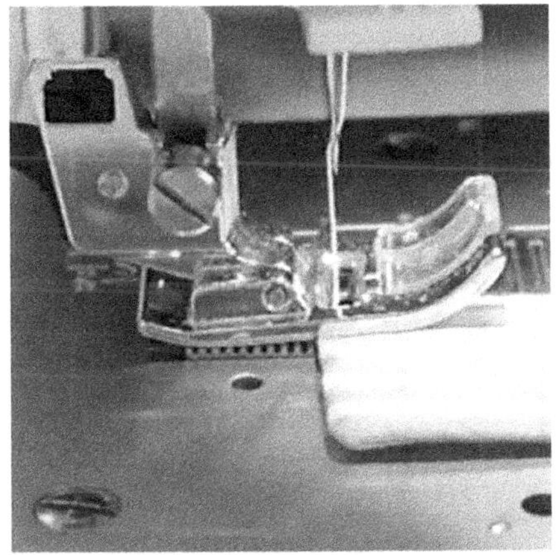

 Place the button at the two ends of the strip and hand sew it on the strip

Hook to your mask

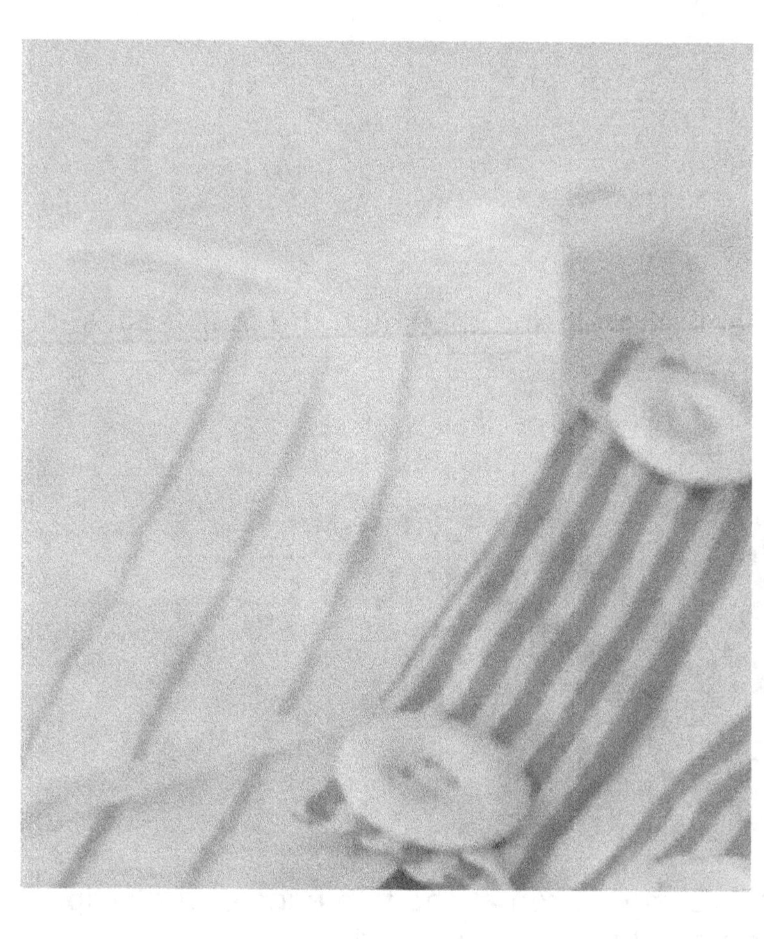

Ways to sterilize and clean your medical face mask

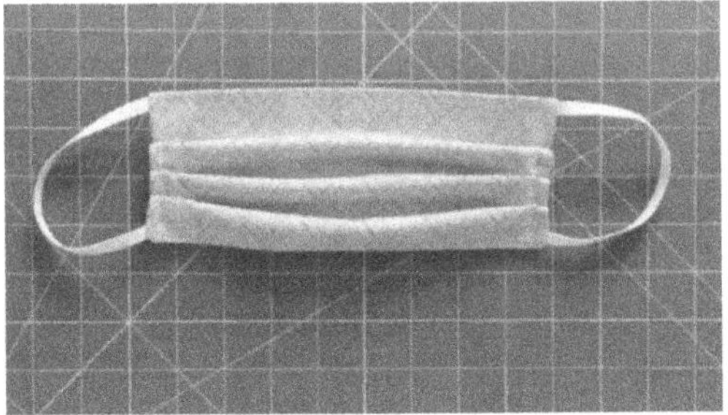

You can reuse your face mask, if you know how to properly sterilize and clean it and if you are not sick already also and you are not a health worker.

First method
Soak it in a hot water of 100 degree Celsius for 10 mins and then using a soft brush gently brush the inside and outside and scrub gently

Then rinse it and rinse with a warm water allow to dry. it is as good as new

Second method
This is for your cloth mask and the N95 mask

Place the mask in a paper bag and then place it in a glass or metal dish and bake at 165-degree F or 70 degree Celsius for 30 minutes Steamed i. then check the temperature with a gun if you have one. it is good again for 5 cycles

Third method

 In this method an Instant Pot Autoclave is used

Place wire rack inside of the pot and place a metal or glass bowl on top of it then put your mask inside the glass or metal bowl. do not add any liquid. Run on manual pressure mode for 5 minutes.

Fourth method

Place the mask in a UVC light box for 20 minutes per side. ensure that the bag is fully zipped, before turning the light on to protect your eyes. with this method the mask can be reused for almost 20 times

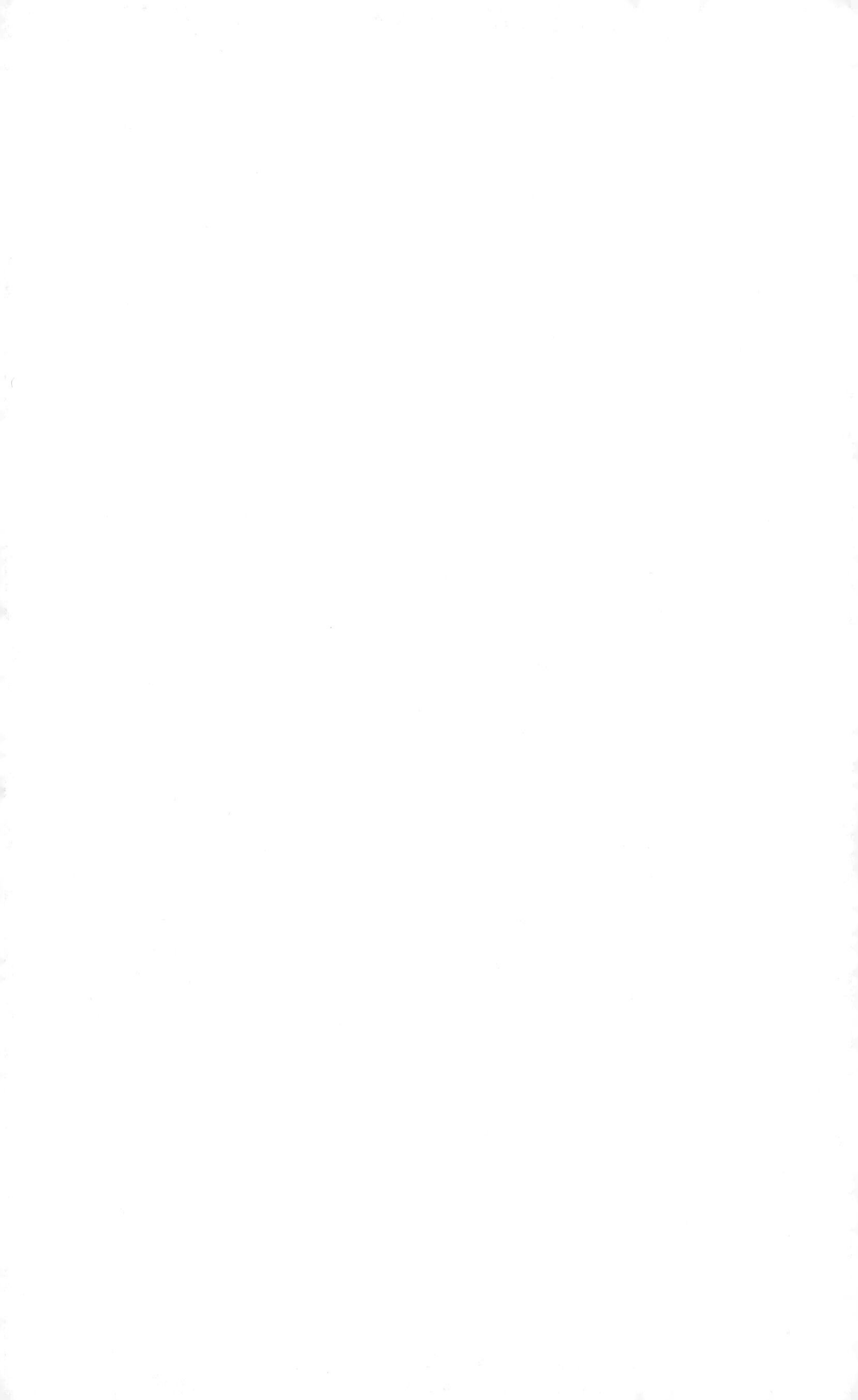

www.ingramcontent.com/pod-product-compliance
Lightning Source LLC
Chambersburg PA
CBHW072126150726
47999CB00005B/2153